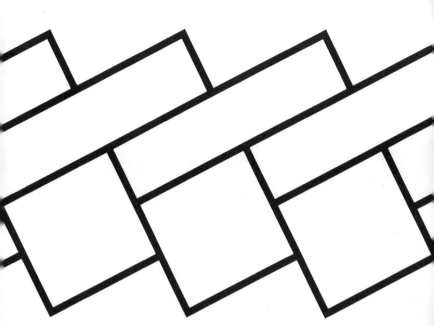

BUILDING
MARKET STRENGTH
THROUGH DRGs

by LEE F. BLOCK
and CHRISTOPHER E. PRESS

Library of Congress Catalog Card Number:
85-62636

International Standard Book Number:
0–931028–73–6

Pluribus Press, Division of Teach'em, Inc.
160 East Illinois Street
Chicago, Illinois 60611

Printed in the United States of America

Acknowledgments

The authors acknowledge the considerable support of their colleagues, including Jacquelyn K. Hirt, Director of Public Relations, John Korte, Director of Corporate Planning, Daniel P. Hogan, Vice President, Treasurer, of St. Francis-St. George Health Services in Cincinnati for their ideas and comments. And Peggy Hedrick, Department Manager, Administrative Support Group, for her support in preparing the manuscript. Special thanks go to William Copeland, President, St. Francis-St. George Health Services. And a special thanks to Jacquelin Weisman. And our families.

All figures presented in this book, with the exception of cited statistics, are hypothetical but drawn from experience to create a point. Any relationship to the experience of a particular institution is entirely coincidental. All figures are masked to protect the source.

Contents

Introduction

This book is written for healthcare marketers, chief executive officers in hospitals, chief financial officers, hospital trustees, medical staffs, and nursing administrators. One could argue that every manager in a hospital clinical setting should take the time to read and understand this book. It could be the key — and certainly one of the keys — to the future financial viability of the institution whether that hospital be a large, tertiary, teaching medical center or a community hospital. Every size institution is and will be affected by DRGs for a long time, even though they may fade as a reimbursement device. This work provides a sound and practical approach to being paid by diagnosis.

The concept of DRGs appears simple enough. Experience shows the *use* of DRGs is more complicated, intricate, and controversial. Physicians complain that in many instances it is difficult to arrive at a diagnosis; hospitals complain that the payments for specific DRGs are inadequate; the government complains that healthcare costs too much; employers complain that their employee coverage is not yet on a DRG system so that their costs can be contained; and patients complain because they leave the hospital too soon to recover at home. Through it all, though, there is a thread of logic. If hospitals and physicians work on the basis of treating an illness or disease, then being paid on the basis of a diagnosis makes sense.

But we're compelled to make one observation. Any instrument as powerful — and quite simply as *present* in a hospital — as DRGs must be understood for its marketing dimension.

In consumer and industrial settings, where tangible products are produced, the marketer pays infinite attention to the design, place, product, and price the marketplace will sustain. In a service setting the "product" is always elusive and abstract. With DRGs the federal government has made specific the products hospitals produce. This is the marketing dimension of DRGs which we have explored — and, we hope, mined some useful findings. This book provides a clear course for the hospital CEO or marketing executive interested in becoming product specific. It demonstrates how to focus that effort.

In a very real sense, hospital managers and trustees need to understand the thrust being presented here, for they will be asked to deal with the services and units in the hospital that require a policy decision concerning their viability. Senior administrators, medical staffs and boards must deal realistically with the services that are financial losers. To keep them, to trade them with nearby institutions for services your institution can provide more efficiently, or to simply close them down — these and others are not simple issues, but they must be dealt with at the highest levels.

Although this is primarily a marketing book, it rests heavily on the foundation of accurate cost accounting in the hospital. (We believe that marketing issues are inseparable from finance issues.) This has long been a subject of diversity and controversy. Here, there must be the now-talked-about "bias for action." Repeatedly we warn that the profitability or loss on a specific DRG has its roots in accurate cost determination. We have no quick remedies for this problem — we warn that hospitals without cost accounting systems that are as accurate as possible will find DRGs and the application of marketing techniques not merely a puzzle but an impossibility. Hospital finance people have labored long and hard in the cost accounting garden. Now they must reap what they have sowed — or begin laboring and sowing in a hurry.

We take no position on the amount of money paid for each DRG or combination of DRGs. The purpose here is to open a window of examination that uses DRGs as products the hospital (and eventually the physician) manages. It makes sense for hospitals to apply the marketing knowledge they are quickly learning to the products they now produce. And to understand the bottom-line impact of successful marketing. This is not judgmental; making money isn't, for the purpose of this book, good, bad or inconse-.quential. But we insist that ignorance of profitability or unprofitability is inexcusable.

There is a serious disclaimer that needs mention here. We are two professional healthcare marketers who see a powerful opportunity for hospitals to take the DRG fact and turn it into a profitable, useful and rewarding instrument. The shortcomings of DRGs are legion, but we see too many executives using these defects as an excuse not to act. The aphorism "half a loaf is better than none" applies. Our perception is that the environment has changed. Period. We view ours as a single approach to the situation. There are others. But, historically the hospital industry has been a reactive one. That is, hospitals have not created major sociological and economic formats for Americans to examine and accept or reject. DRGs were not created by hospitals, they were created by an external force. This book presents a positive agenda to meet that creation.

CHAPTER 1

The third answer is up to you

The hospital has long been tagged the doctor's workshop. Authors, depending on their viewpoint, variously described doctors as noble scholars methodically working in a sophisticated laboratory, or stunted elves expensively tinkering. Whatever your politics, the basic description is — was — correct. The hospital supplied the wares for physicians to construct repairs on broken people. It worked marvelously. Hospitals provided the capital, the labor, and the organization. Physicians provided professional skill and patients.

Sophisticated, civilized and gruesomely expensive. Because in a very workshop-like way, every job was custom-built. Each patient was treated as a unique chore, and a specifically-designed and constructed hospital stay was engineered by the physician for each patient. No different than a custom-built car, home, piece of furniture, or suit, the economic rules that applied were no different; when it's made to your order, it is going to be expensive.

DRGs have changed all this. No custom medicine.

No custom cars, homes, furniture, or suits. 470 varieties. Economy through standardization and, naturally, compromise.

The immediate consequences are at least three. First is an intensified wrestling match for control of the hospital's product. Do physicians control it, as they have historically? Or does hospital management? An important question for a marketer. Second, now that there are standard units — or products — how can we better understand them and apply proven marketing techniques? Third, since standardization means compromise (in terms of product features), where will the market tolerate compromise? What features can be amended without alienating the buyers?

The first question we hope will be answered with management. Clearly, control of the hospital must be in concert with physicians and other professionals, but management must have the final word. (If for no other reason than the courts have held the board liable for what occurs, and management is present to fulfill the policies and directives of the board.) The second question will be answered, we hope, in the course of this book. The third question, unfortunately, you'll have to answer for yourself.

DRGs unquestionably have become a useful system for classifying patients. This taxonomy can be used for reimbursement. It can be used for medical research. But, most importantly for the marketer, it can be used to understand what's happening in the organization and the marketplace.

In an earlier day the question might have been posed, "What kind of patients are we treating?" The answers would have been many. One person might have said, "Dr. Smith, the cardiologist, is our number one admitter — therefore we must do a lot of cardiac work." Another might have said, "The Jones Group — family practice — has three of the top five admitters. We must have a big family practice business." The point is that there was no common language. No universal system. All measures were proxies.

Today, you know exactly what you're doing because you can count discharges according to each DRG. More importantly, you can trace physicians, events in the hospital, labor, supplies — virtually everything — to a DRG. From the standpoint of information, management, and control, this is nothing short of a revolution.

Typically, managers lack clinical backgrounds and therefore have little comprehension of how DRGs were constructed. A deeply technical understanding isn't required, but an overview to acquaint managers with certain major issues which may affect using DRGs in a marketing context is important.

DRGs were developed for the federal government as a utilization review mechanism. They are not the first such classification system invented nor are they the only such system. DRGs are drawn from previous generations of classification techniques.

Patients were once classified according to the principal diagnosis. Clearly, such a broad system would give little guidance to any user: UR, marketing, finance, or operations. Physician practice patterns alone — the way they might phrase the patient diagnosis — could distort data.

The Commission on Professional and Hospital Activities (CPHA) developed the second system. Here, all patient diagnoses were organized into 349 mutually exclusive major diagnosis categories. Sounds manageable so far. However, each major diagnosis category was subdivided:

- presence/absence of secondary diagnosis
- presence/absence of surgery
- five age cohorts

This produced approximately 7,000 patient classes.

ICD-9-CM elaborated on the work of CPHA. The International Classification of Diseases, Ninth Revision, Clinical Modification was also developed for utilization, quality, and peer review application. It relies on 398 diagnosis groups, and is subdivided somewhat like CPHA. The byproduct is 7,960 outcomes.

DRGs were developed in the late 60's through mid-70's at Yale University. Since then, several generations have come and gone before the one we know today, which has 23 Major Diagnosis Categories (MDC) and 467 groupings.

The MDCs generally mirror major organ systems, except for a few cases (such as injury, poisoning, and toxic effects of drugs) where impractical. Though used for Medicare reimbursement, the DRG system of classifying applies to patients of all ages.

OTHER SYSTEMS OF CLASSIFICATION

DRGs are not the only system available to classify inpatient activity.

Disease staging is a system of organizing patients

THE THIRD ANSWER IS UP TO YOU | 9

according to their transit through the varying stages of severity and disease. It is most commonly associated with cancer, but is attributed to John Fathergill in 1748.

Others include Patient Management Categories, VA Multi-Level Care Groups, AS-SCORE (A = age of patient; S = systems, i.e. organs involved; S = stage of disease; CO = complications; RE = response to therapy), Severity of Illness Index, MD-DADO (Physician Discharge Abstract Data Optimal System) and Generic Algorithms. Medical records professionals could explain the functions of these systems, none of which lends itself to a marketing purpose as readily as DRGs.

WEAKNESSES OF DRGs

DRGs aren't flawless. In development for a decade, drawn from dormant data, they are found to have vulnerabilities. Among the major ones:

- They do not appropriately account for the severity of illness (the loss of a patient's function) or intensity of service (the comparative volumes of services used in management of the case).

- They only mimic current therapeutic practice. They are not a norm or an optimum.

- They derive from dormant and conceivably inconsistent or inaccurate data (discharge summaries).

- They only apply to inpatient care.

These weaknesses do have relevance for the marketing application.

SEVERITY/INTENSITY is the most common criticism from those who argue for more reimbursement. Every hospital manager believes his patients are sicker than the norm. Therefore, they use more service which merits more reimbursement. If this proves true, there are cost implications which may now be depressing profitability.

DRGs MIMIC PRESENT PRACTICE. This is the least understood, and in some respects, most controversial drawback. DRGs are only an "averaging" of current — not optimal — practice. Again, this has implications in physician recruitment/retirement, and will be discussed in Chapter 3. Also, it means that DRGs will be amended over time to adjust for medical technology.

The *ORIGINS IN DORMANT DATA* argument is a weak one. Laws of large numbers, probability, sampling theory, and other statistical science rules argue that, overall, there is material accuracy in the DRG system. The inaccuracies are so far outnumbered by valid findings that they have no important effect on the outcome. There is an opportunity for hospital-specific error in data collection and classification. Incorrectly coded charts, improperly written discharge summaries and other vagaries could cause a hospital to report an errant number of discharges in a DRG. This is an issue for the manager in collecting, reviewing and evaluating data. However, because a facility's revenue depends upon accurate summaries and coding, most hospitals have moved very quickly to teach physicians the best way to summarize, and to insure capable employees perform the codings. Gaming the system for optimal reimbursement probably poses as great a risk as coding error.

That DRGs apply only to *INPATIENT CARE* is a

transient condition. They'll soon be applied to outpatient and physician care. Conceivably, they will be applied per patient per incident, and the reimbursement sum will have to be shared among physicians, inpatient provider, outpatient provider, home care provider, pharmacist, therapists, and so on.

DRGs are complex in their origin and clinical application. They are also complex as a reimbursement device. As we will see, they are a technological quantum leap for hospital marketing managers, but still complex. While marketers must know the major structural premises of DRGs, the specific nuances from both the clinical and reimbursement viewpoints for marketing purposes are less important. We can't amend the discharge summaries, or ICD-9-CM. We can't amend the assigned wage weight index for our region. But we can change the way we think about marketing hospital services. Remember that DRGs:

- give us something against which we can assign and manage costs and predictable prices,

- make individual compendium prices for services meaningless,

- make cost centers where there once were revenue centers,

- create enormous pressure for "cookbook medicine",

- create a need for a new marketing information system,

- provide something we can finally call a product, against which, in turn, all marketing principles can be applied.

CHAPTER 2

Revenue centers have become cost centers

Costs and prices aren't the same thing. They never have been, but in a cost-plus era it was easy enough to get confused. Price equalled the cost plus a standard percentage. Managers who think costs and prices are the same will run into trouble under DRGs. *Costs* are outlays an organization incurs to get its products to market. *Prices* are what it hopes to receive from buyers. *Profit* occurs when the organization succeeds. This presents a very fundamental change in hospital thinking.

In most cases, financial officers have no trouble getting this straight. If they are smart, and concerned, they'll make sure that everyone they know in the hospital has this straight. This can be done with mini conferences or with memos, or both. The incentives for reducing costs and reducing length of stay must be explicit and clear to all.

Under cost-plus, a hospital has thousands of prices, from the room charge to a 4" × 4" sterile gauze pad to half-an-hour of OR time. Under cost-plus systems, there is always the incentive to increase activity. This is axiomatic. It is equally axiomatic that under DRGs, this incentive evaporates. It should be replaced by an incentive to reduce activity and unit cost; however, this does not uniformly occur.

In any event, under cost-plus and other non-DRG systems, a patient's bill is the accumulation of prices associated with discrete units of service. A chest X-ray, a CBC, a myleogram, or other specific services. With a DRG system, a lump-sum payment is made, and service decisions effectively reduce the beginning and continuing balance.

It might help non-accountants to picture a patient as having been given Monopoly money by the insurer upon entry to your facility. $3600, say. Everytime a service is rendered, payment is made. At the end of the stay, the cashier is given the balance. Clearly, every ancillary service department, nursing, and all departments are cost centers.

For example:

Receipts from Pt 12345,

DRG XYZ, $3083.00

Day 1 Deductions	−$755 =	$2328
Day 2 Deductions	− 758 =	1570
Day 3 Deductions	− 445 =	1125
Day 4 Deductions, discharge	− 398 =	727
Balance	$727	

It makes no sense whatever to use compendium prices as the figure for calculating deductions, except to obtain a gross comparison between pre- and post-DRG reimbursements. Because of the vagaries of cost-plus reimbursement, however, one could easily tally a sum of charges against a DRG which would substantially exceed the DRG rate.

DRG 127

REIMBURSEMENT	$XXXX
AVERAGE CHARGES BY CATEGORY	
NURSING, ROUTINE CARE	$ 1181
NURSING, SPECIAL CARE	1021
SUPPLIES	433
ANCILLARY (X-RAY, NUC. MED, INHALATION)	1123
PHARMACY	729
MISCELLANEOUS	201
TOTAL	$4688

What does one do with the answer? If the total exceeds reimbursement, it's a safe bet that nothing's changed. If you were losing money, you probably still are. If you were making money, you probably still are. If volume hasn't changed. If costs haven't changed. If you *knew* whether you were making or losing money. On the whole, you can see it provides little guidance.

The only relevant numbers to be deducted from the price are the costs associated with "manufacturing" the DRG, and only certain of them. This will be discussed in detail in the next chapter.

We hope it is evident to you that the prices on discrete services are no longer meaningful for DRG-reimbursed inpatients. This can cause confusion and stress among managers who deliver service. The radiology and lab managers, for example, were once the organizational heroes — major revenue centers. Now they play a pivotal role in managing costs. The behaviors required are very different, and though it exceeds the typical marketing manager's purview to control these managers, he or she must know, and in some cases, champion this new perspective. The fewer tests or the fewer X-rays, the more money the hospital makes. It used to be the other way around.

The purpose here is not to debate the moral, ethical, and related issues which arise as a byproduct of these changed incentives. The facts speak for themselves. The old incentive was to spend. Everybody did, and it was too expensive. The new incentive is to control costs. Right or wrong, that's the way it is.

But in the rush to control costs, it's worthwhile to note that there are different kinds of costs, with different degrees of importance for marketers. There are four major kinds of costs.

Four cost functions

All managers, not only CFOs must understand four cost functions in order to appropriately allocate resources and accurately assess the profitability of a DRG. The four cost functions are:

- Fixed
- Semi-Fixed
- Variable
- Semi-Variable

FIXED costs are just that: fixed. Irrespective of the organization's output, these costs are unchanged. Examples include rent, interest, and depreciation. Hospitals are known as high-fixed cost organizations because of the expensive technology, the buildings, and large labor requirements.

SEMI-FIXED costs change with output, but not directly. Examples include labor and certain utilities. For example, a certain number of full-time equivalents (FTEs) can accommodate a range of output between 100-200 units of service. Output consistently above 200 units would cause labor to be added, increasing costs.

Fixed and semi-fixed costs are often called indirect costs since they do not directly stem from producing a unit of service. Fixed and semi-fixed costs are not to be mistaken for uncontrollable or permanent costs. They can be reduced or eliminated.

VARIABLE costs are directly correlated to output. At zero output, there are zero variable costs. Examples include medical supplies and pharmaceuticals. Hospitals have relatively low variable costs.

SEMI-VARIABLE costs vary with output above a certain baseline. Dietary services are examples of such costs. The entire kitchen must be in place, at a baseline, but patient meals vary with output (census). Variable and semi-variable costs are often called direct costs since they stem directly from producing a unit.

The implications of being high-fixed-cost, low-variable-cost are not always apparent at first. The concept of contribution margin sheds light. It holds that the sales dollar ultimately has to pay the direct costs (variable and semi-variable) of providing the product, and the indirect (fixed and semi-fixed) costs of providing the product. It also focuses on the next unit of output to be produced: the so-called marginal or incremental unit. The contribution margin is simply calculated: CM = Price — Variable Costs. In some cases, it is useful to express the contribution as a ratio of variable cost to price. This is the contribution ratio.

Note that the direct costs are those traceable to the specific incremental unit produced. Indirect costs are those which must be paid irrespective of the decision to produce (or not produce) the incremental unit.

FIXED COSTS

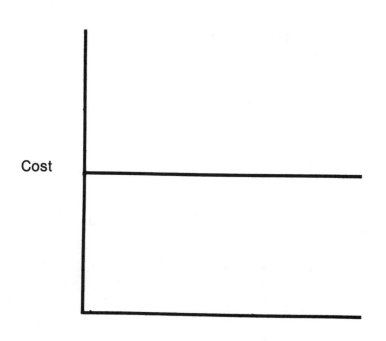

Examples:

Depreciation

Interest

Rent

Lease

SEMI-FIXED COSTS

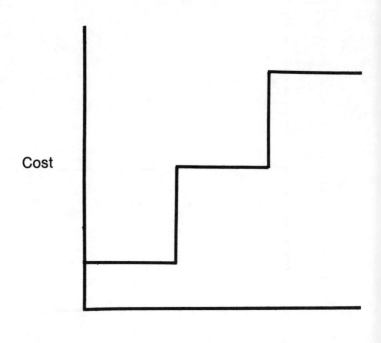

Output

Examples:

Salaries

Fringe Ben◄

Utility Cost◄

VARIABLE COSTS

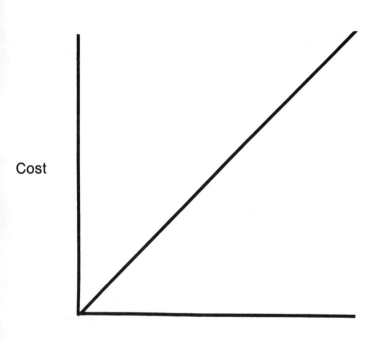

Cost

Output

Examples:

Medical Supplies

Pharmaceuticals

SEMI-VARIABLE COSTS

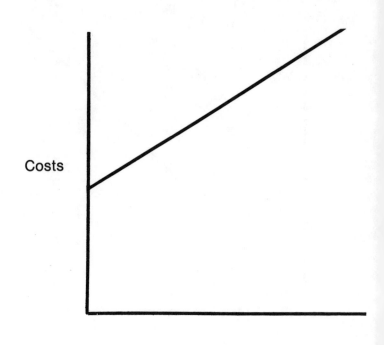

Costs

Output

Examples:

Maintenan
Services

Housekee

Dietary Se

For example, let's say that DRG 127 in your hospital is reimbursed by all payors at $3,500. Your hospital is operating efficiently and profitably. So far this year you've seen 400 cases of DRG 127. On the 401st patient, how much incremental expense will you endure? Probably very little — food, radiology supplies, medical and lab supplies, drugs, housekeeping and linens, no labor or plant. The incremental cost may only be several hundred dollars, leaving a balance of, say, $2,800 to contribute to other expenses. What are the incentives with respect to DRG 127? To sustain volume at the very least, and ideally increase volume.

In this case, the contribution margin is ($3500-$700) = $2800. The contribution ratio is (price - variable cost)/price = $2800/3500 = 80 per cent.

Not every accounting system captures variable costs and calculates contribution margin. Some financial managers and others use fully allocated costing which restates the costs associated with the next unit of output. These techniques vary, but some simply take average costs as derived from total costs divided by total output. Everything is included in the costs: rent (allocated per square foot usually), labor (including a fraction of management's time), etc. All direct and indirect costs are part of the calculations. Watch how the analysis can change.

TOTAL COSTS TO PRODUCE DRG 127: $2,100,000

AVERAGE COST/UNIT AT "X" OUTPUT	
300	$ 7,000
400	$ 5,250
500	$ 4,200
600	$ 3,500

The finance officer, in good faith, would contend that the 401st unit lost $1,750 for the organization, and that the product will not break-even until the 601st unit. He or she would accuse the marketing department of being careless with numbers.

In the sense that all costs must be paid, that view is infallibly correct. In the analysis, however, the benefits of that many patients, regardless of what the 401st does to the statistics, are ignored. If you can sell something for more than it directly costs you to produce it, all other things being equal, *sell.* Any funds over and above the variable costs contribute to fixed costs, and ultimately profit.

EXAMPLES

Because, as it was noted, hospitals have such high fixed costs and low variable costs, it is almost unimaginable that a hospital would have a negative contribution margin on a particular DRG. The profitability problem facing some hospitals stems from excessive fixed costs — or the other side of the coin, low volume.

High fixed cost, low variable cost organizations live and die by volume. Or the lack of it. When volume falls, fixed costs must be adjusted. Automakers are useful examples. During the recession of the early 80's, automobile sales volume plummeted. Losses soared, because of the monstrous fixed costs. To remedy the problem: plants were closed, blue collar labor laid off, white collar labor fired by the tens of thousands, and so on. The outcome is that a lower total volume of sales is required to reach a profit.

Units Sold	×	Contribution Margin	−	Fixed Costs	=	Profit (Loss)
100,000	×	$50		7,000,000		(2,000,000)
				5,000,000		-0-
				4,000,000		1,000,000

If volume cannot be increased, costs must be reduced.

For a hospital marketing manager, certain lessons emerge. Admissions are not increasing. That is, volume is flat. To sustain volume means sustaining market share; to increase volume means stealing market share, an expensive and often grueling ordeal.

Predictions of the continued boom in the Gray Market, perhaps large enough to create overall market growth, are exciting but uncertain. Inpatient volumes may be cannabilized (an unfortunate marketing term when used in a hospital context) by alternate delivery systems.

In the final analysis: again, it's improbable that a DRG lacks some contribution value. However, volume must be maintained. This is a clear and key marketing duty and objective. Fixed costs must be controlled by senior management. Variable costs must be managed to provide an optimal contribution margin.

CONTROLLING VARIABLE COSTS

There are two facets to variable costs: the cost of the resource(s), and the amount of resource(s) used (volume). In a manufacturing context, only the former item is an issue since the latter is standardized, or becomes linked to product differentiation in the market. For example, again, automobiles. The cost of the input is carefully controlled. The amount of resources going into a vehicle, once into production, is precisely predictable, and difference among vehicles relate to product differences. In a hospital, it's very different.

Costs

The first contrast between a hospital and other process manufacturers is that a hospital operates all of its production lines simultaneously and in the same space. A manufacturer tools for a certain product, manufactures the desired quantity, then retools for the next product. On it goes. This obviously could never happen in a hospital. And it means that certain production lines are standing by and costs accrue even though they are idle, and others are very busy. Crossover among tasks is the goal to reduce the level of standby costs, thereby reducing semi-variable costs.

The most important variable costs within management's unilateral control are: labor, which may be 50 per cent to 60 per cent of total expenses, and supplies, which are the second leading category at 13-18 per cent.

Labor is most variable on nursing units where there

is the ability to more accurately predict need. Admissions are typically known (except through the emergency department), the acuity of patients can be assessed, and staffing can be adjusted. In other units, it is often more difficult to control because volume can't be predicted and the service can't be warehoused. For instance, it is difficult to predict day-to-day CT scan volume. So, a technician must be present. His or her ability to perform other duties becomes important, as noted above.

Supplies are an enormous cost for a hospital. Whereas labor is typically a semi-variable cost, supplies more closely resemble pure variable costs. For an average facility — 300 beds — the cost may total $10,000,000. Certain supplies are linked to physician order, and they'll be discussed below. But others are not. They are consumed or conserved according to the discretion of 1000 employees.

For example, the radiographer who must frequently repeat examinations because of poor training, defective equipment, inferior film, etc., imposes a distinct additional cost. At $3.00 or $5.00 per sheet of silver coated plastic, accuracy has value.

Another example is controlling what becomes contaminated by patient contact. Keeping supplies distant from patients until needed helps insure that unneeded supplies aren't wasted.

These may seem minor, but the cumulative effect is substantial. A 5 per cent improvement liberates $500,000 to be supplied to fixed costs and profit.

Physician-driven variable costs

As we know, much activity occurs as a result of physician orders. Because these orders are related to an admission, they are by definition variable costs. They can be traced to a particular patient. Controlling the resources a physician applies to a patient becomes critical, and can call for some savvy demarketing.

For example, imagine a high admitter (200 per year) who has a summary profile as follows as compared to the other physicians in the department.

	Physician	*Department*
LENGTH OF STAY (L.O.S.)	9.5 days	6.8 days
X-RAY EXAMS/ PATIENT	4.4	2.5
LAB TESTS/PATIENT	8.1	5.0
PHYSICAL THERAPY HOURS/PATIENT	2.7	1.1
OTHER ANCILLARY/ EXAMS/PATIENT	15.4	10.9

This physician causes you, in some measure, to:

- overstaff nursing to accommodate the extra days of service

- over inventory and over use radiology supplies

- overstaff laboratory and over use laboratory supplies (and perhaps pathology)

- overstaff and overuse PT

Again, the effect is probably not that the physician is unprofitable. But this behavior reduces contribution margin in certain ways, which forces volume to go higher in order to cover fixed costs and earn a profit.

The hospital can calculate the resources used by physicians in the care of patients by DRG. These can be presented tabularly or graphically to demonstrate those physicians who exceed the averages. When those physicians are confronted with their patterns, they typically reply "my patients are sicker" or "those other doctors aren't being prudently thorough." In the first case, it's unlikely that a physician has attracted a clientele of patients who demonstrate legitimate epidemiological abberations from a normal population. Laws of large numbers and random sampling simply make it improbable. In the second case, recall that we mentioned a criticism of DRGs is that they aren't an optimum — they merely represent current practice, right, wrong or indifferent. That deflates this — and most every other argument — in defense of overutilization.

These responses can be explained to and accepted by most physicians — but we don't recommend the sledge-hammer touch in discussing such issues.

Having traced resources used by DRG by physician, the next step to attach costs to those resources.

Costs of resources

There are two techniques for this process. One is to use a ratio of costs to charges (RCC). In this technique, a coefficient is applied against charges to determine approximate cost. Again, the cost is ideally the variable cost, but for most facilities it will include other costs.

The second approach depends upon more thorough cost accounting analysis to measure, rather than estimate, costs. This approach is much more expensive, time-consuming, and difficult. It cannot be said often enough that the accurate discovery of costs is a crucial step in DRG marketing. The organization must know its margins in order to know where to place its marketing effort, or to know where its market's preferences are costing money.

The goal is a report which demonstrates the following summary information, whether attained through approximation (risky) or direct assessment.

DRG #88 - CHRONIC OBSTRUCTIVE PULMONARY DISEASE

Physician #	# Cases	Average Variable Cost	Price	Average Contribution Margin
231	10	381	—	2739
234	8	366		2754
240	7	401	3120	2719
245	8	181		2939
247	13	359		2761
699	1	752	—	2368
	47	349	3120	2771

AVG VARIABLE COSTS PER DISCHARGE, BY PHYSICIAN, COMPARED TO PRICE, DRG 88, 1Q85

This graph demonstrates several things. First, it shows information regarding DRG 88 for the first quarter of 1985, during which time six physicians discharged 47 patients in this DRG. Physicians 231, 234,

240 and 247 are driving the average. Physician 245 is of keen interest, since the variable costs on eight patients averaged half of the group average. These questions come to mind:

Is there a data collection error?

Are patients being slighted with inferior care?

Are the other physicians over-intensive?

Does he or she know or do something that would cause the other physicians to reduce their average variable charges to the same level?

Did he or she "get lucky" and have some "easy" patients?

Did he or she perform certain examinations in an outpatient setting before admitting the patient?

The list goes on.

Physician 699 was "zapped." One patient and high costs. This is also of interest. First, it is evident from the number that the department is different from the others. (Say, family practice versus pulmonary medicine.) So he or she may not be as skilled in reaching a COPD diagnosis. We can also tell by the number that this is a new staff member, and probably young. If Dr. 699 continues to admit to this DRG, we would likely acquaint him or her with the methods of Dr. 240. If findings on Dr. 245 prove positive, introduce the two of them to one another!

At this time there is an important point to be made. Let no reader — physician or administrator — feel that the book overlooks the strong need for physician participation in marketing DRGs or the physician involvement with the process suggested here.

Physicians need to know the thrust of what is being done and proposed in the marketing of DRGs. There is no intention of keeping it a secret from the medical staff. They need to know and understand.

Moreover, the medical staff — physician to physician — can be the most effective method of making important changes in individual physician behavior within a given DRG.

As the case just mentioned indicates, Doctor 699 may be new on the staff and may need to be introduced to Dr. 240. If the latter knows the objective of bringing Dr. 699 into the average for DRG 88, he or she had better have the ammunition and information concerning the DRG and Dr. 699's overuse.

Above all, healthcare marketers need to be sensitive to the issues involved in any DRG over-use. It's more useful and much more effective if a physician talks to a physician about such matters. For a layman to discuss use and over-use of various integral parts of a DRG may be difficult — not impossible, but difficult.

Another note. Such a graph is constructed using standards and averages and therefore portrays an approximation of events, not a description of a precise event. Standards are built during the cost-finding process, so that it is known that the standard chest X-ray has a variable cost of $X. In the course of events, experience will vary around this standard, both above and below. But the standard is the expected, usually attainable outcome. From here, an assessment is made of the standard number of chest X-rays for DRG 88: COPD. In this manner, we have the standard variable cost for chest X-rays for DRG 88. The same logic is applied for the other variable cost items within the DRG.

Clinical professionals fault this process, citing an exceptionally wide distribution of outcomes, not neat, compact bell curves. There is some merit to the criticism but, as we've said, such criticisms are not a legitimate excuse for foregoing the analysis.

COOKBOOK MEDICINE

Why should one physician regularly consume twice the resources that others do? Or, why should one physician regularly consume half the resources? Can't there be a standard protocol for each DRG?

As managers, we depend upon standardization to conserve our time, energy, effort and money. We prepare standard reports. Standard budgets, where we only focus on exceptions. Even such subjective processes as long range planning can be routinized into discrete steps.

In the finest restaurants, meals are prepared according to a standard. In quick-service restaurants, the same is true. Portions are controlled. Waste and spoilage are controlled and monitored. Why not have a cookbook for DRG 88?

That's a rhetorical question. However, for the organization that can identify and negotiate with efficient physicians, there are tremendous opportunities. Assume you discover that DRG 294 — diabetes greater than age 36 — has very low variable costs and a high contribution margin. Admissions are coming from a group of young physicians who are talented, but still getting started in their practice.

You are now able to package DRG 294 for direct sale to industry, insurers and alternate providers. You have a combination of unique selling points, price and physician ability among them. You aren't compelled to price the product at the Medicare rate — it can be higher or lower. And you aren't compelled to solicit business in every DRG. You can be selective, and attack competitors' vulnerabilities and/or market vacuums.

Cookbooks? Not necessarily. But you can give the buyer a specification detail which indicates the standard protocols for DRG 294, and the conditions which prompt outliers. Buyers can then compare this to their own current utilization patterns, with the expectation of your hospital coming out ahead.

All of this depends, however, upon accurate and extensive data collection.

The most important thing to keep in mind here is the desired outcome: to make the individual physician involved understand and accept the need to modify the way tests and other care for specific patients are ordered. The manner in which this is accomplished will depend on the institution and the medical staff organization. Ideally, of course, the medical staff should undertake this kind of review on a regular basis. The administration can help by ensuring that the medical staff has the necessary mechanism and information for doing this. Some may say another "committee" won't do it, and maybe it won't. But some mechanism needs to be established.

Red lights do not have to flash and whistles need not blow when a physician goes outside certain DRG guidelines. But the medical staff must show an awareness of the need for cost containment and prudence in ordering tests for patients. Regular meetings between physicians who work consistently within the guidelines and those who routinely fall within the outlier category can help achieve this goal.

It is dangerous for administrators to move into this area. They risk accusation of interfering with the practice of medicine. It is safer and more effective for the medical staff to act on behalf of the administration.

The smart administrator keeps the objective in clear focus — modification of physician behavior — and finds a way to get the job done through the medical staff, not around it.

Placement agencies are full of the vitae of administrators who tried to do all of this themselves without regard to the sensitive nature of the task and the long term harm they could cause. Bringing physicians into a norm for each profitable DRG should be viewed as part of a system, not as a series of bandages applied only in emergency situations.

KEY POINTS

In most industries, the cost to produce a unit of service is known in advance with reasonable certainty. In those cases where it isn't known, management can commit or withdraw effort without moral consequence. In hospitals, the cost isn't known in advance, and controlling costs can affect human lives. The marketing manager, if reasoned recommendations on how to match organizational ability with market need are to be reached, must have accurate cost information. In most cases, one will have to be a protagonist to get it. The important things to remember are:

- do not look at your historical prices for these services,

- do look at direct variable costs,

- do focus on contribution margin.

The desired measure is direct variable cost per unit of service. For example, the direct costs for DRG 127, heart failure and shock, are, on average $850. Given reimbursement of $3800, this leaves $2950 as a contribution margin. In cases such as this you have no problems. Or do you? If your competition receives the same reimbursement, but can get costs down to $750, there's a strong incentive to solicit more business — and perhaps one of your physicians. Controlling unit costs is important to control your competitive position.

INFORMATION SYSTEMS

DRGs are forcing an overhaul in marketing information collection and management. It is not a retooling of current data systems as much as inventing completely new files.

There are an infinite number of possible data tabulations for DRGs. Depending upon the institution, the needs will vary. Here are some possible information files:

Per cent of DRG XXX arriving by emergency room, direct admission, scheduled appointment.

Per cent of DRG XXX discharged to home health-care.

Per cent of DRG XXX discharged by MD 1, 2, 3 etc.

Total discharge of DRG XXX.

What is the age distribution of DRG XXX patients?

What is the income distribution of DRG XXX patients?

What is the bad debt distribution of DRG XXX patients?

What is the education distribution of DRG XXX patients?

What is the sex distribution of DRG XXX patients?

What is the variable cost per DRG?

What are the resources consumed by each DRG?

Which DRGs are discharged to:
other hospitals?
home health?
nursing homes?
home?

Who were the insurers for DRG XXX?

Who were the employers for DRG XXX?

What were the DRGs for patients of ages X to Y?

What were the DRGs for patients of incomes X to Y?

What were the DRGs for patients of zip code X to Y?

CHAPTER 4

Ordering the product line

Earlier we contended that the marketing posture in a healthcare setting begs for product. In all service organizations the product, in a marketing sense, is difficult to pin-down and make specific. The marketer is most effective when a product, a service, an object, a "thing" is the subject of marketing know-how.

The healthcare setting has been abstract (until now) for the marketer. The search for the thing in healthcare to be marketed has led to the obstetrics department, or the burn unit, or the emergency room or the long list of other abstractions that have been taken to the marketplace. One should add here that the marketer in health has registered some resounding successes, not-withstanding the difficulty found in the programs developed with a lack of substance — a product. The contention here is that DRGs provide the long elusive products we have been searching to find. Consider — DRG 127 — it has form and matter. There are shape, form, and product qualities to all of the DRGs.

So now, the marketer, in concert with planners, auditors, cost analysts and the finance department, must begin the hard work. It begins by learning which of the DRGs are high volume. Having discovered this, it's necessary to look at the contribution margins.

For example, the top 20 or 30 DRGs must be found (if not already known) and then cost-finding begins. The outcome should be four general categories:

● High contribution

● Moderate contribution

● Low contribution

● Below-potential contribution

Clearly, this separation gives the marketer the ammunition to produce a marketing program to channel resources where they belong — where they can increase market share, profit, or satisfy some other corporate goal.

Before discussing the possibilities and implications of this thesis, one should be aware of a major pitfall. It is outside the field of marketing, but it is something that marketers and others need to be perfectly aware of and never lose sight of.

This nemesis rests in the cost accounting area. If, indeed, the DRGs we think are profitable are poorly cost designated, our problem will be magnified if we market them. The constant push of hospital accounting people into the accurate cost accounting methodology necessary under the DRG system should not be hindered. Rather, it needs constant stimulation and the allocation of funds to accomplish.

The DRG method of payment for services in hospitals should spur the search and method of cost finding even more. If the search stops short, the DRG payment and our ability to designate which DRGs are profitable will falter; that will mean disaster when it's time for the institution to pay its vendors and employees.

Opinion is divided on this issue, but we hold that the likelihood of a DRG having a negative contribution margin is practically nil. This is true because of the low variable costs of rendering inpatient hospital care. Trying to assess profit by DRG will always prove elusive because it will involve extremely complex, and frequently arbitrary, calculations. For example, how much of the cost of an Astra Analyzer or fluoroscope should be applied against DRG 88? or DRG 127? This is an area of theoretical cost allocation which is extremely controversial.

So we advocate abandoning the concept of profit when looking at DRGs. The relevant concept is contribution margin, and from a managerial standpoint, the goal is *managing* the contribution margin. That's done by managing costs and volumes. And we readily concede that it's easier said than done.

Having ordered the DRGs into these four categories, management should proceed with sustaining, increasing, or revising activity according to circumstances. The regular menu of marketing and management options can now be much more sensibly applied.

For example, there's no reason to promote the below-potential group until they've come closer to their potential. There may be good reason, however, to recruit a physician into a category to increase volume or displace a high-cost practitioner.

We can't say it often enough: in the absence of the

analysis we recommend, implementing programs is akin to gambling. It may pay off. But it may prove ineffective or at cross-purposes with organizational objectives.

Armed with this information and your hospital's strategic plan, you can choose the segments where you want (and are able) to compete. The beauty of this analysis is it presents the opportunity to cease shotgun marketing. Now you can use rifle fire, putting resources where you want them with clear objectives in mind.

There's no question about it. Determining the contribution margin of DRGs must be based on the most modern technology for cost determination. Without a sound cost allocation method in the hospital, the DRG method of payment will eventually put the hospital out of business — and certainly the marketing method of DRGs espoused here will be of little deterrent on that road to oblivion.

The assumption then is that DRG contributions are neither a mirage nor a good guess in a hospital. Rather, they are based on a sensible and meaningful cost allocation method.

An important aside is timely. Who really produces the costs that go into a DRG? That is, who is responsible for the total cost of an individual patient's care? There are two schools of thought as to who produces a DRG's costs: hospital and physician. Like so many "clear cut" issues, the answer lies in between.

Hospitals produce DRG costs in the sense that they provide the necessary labor, supplies, and equipment to act upon physician requests. But, it is the physician request which produces a series of actions which create the end product. So, as always, the physician orders the product and the hospital produces it.

This issue is most relevant since it leads inevitably to one question: Who is responsible for an "unprofitable" or "profitable" DRG? A simple formula helps.

$$\text{TOTAL COST} = \text{UNIT COST} \times \text{UNIT VOLUME}$$

This clarifies the issue beyond question. Management is responsible for unit costs. Physicians, under the view of utilization control and review, are responsible for unit volume. Profitability and unprofitability can be a function of one or both of these variables being askew.

A particular DRG could be unprofitable because a particular physician's practice pattern over-depends upon diagnostic technology. Similarly, it could be unprofitable because the hospital has too high supply or labor costs. To make decisions, management must be able to isolate these variables of unit cost and unit volume.

THE HIGH CONTRIBUTION MARGIN DRGs

Let's look at the DRGs that are high contribution margin. For now we will disregard their complexity or other aspects of their profile. All we need to know is that there is a certain group of DRGs which produce a handsome contribution margin for the hospital.

In any hospital the high contribution margin DRG list will not be extensive. Most hospitals have not examined these DRGs in quite the way being suggested here. They need to be viewed on the basis of which physicians provide the patients with these diagnoses. And once we determine which physicians on our staff they are, we need to encourage their continued and increased admissions of those specific DRGs along current practice patterns.

One specific action here is to identify for the physicians those DRGs of theirs that are high contribution margin. This, if done correctly, should point out the high degree of expertise the physicians and the hospital have achieved in that DRG. And it should make clear how from both the physicians' point of view and that of their patients, delivery of the specific DRG has a high degree of effectiveness. One would hope quality in that delivery is an important component as well.

It is strongly recommended that product managers be appointed for these DRGs. These managers may come from the administrative staff, nursing staff, and other positions already in the hospital. In addition to their regular jobs they become the matrix manager of a group of DRGs. They examine the cost reports for each, analyze each facet of the DRG delivery to see where cost-savings may occur, and manage their DRGs just as though they were products. The objective: raise or sustain the contribution margin without forfeiture of quality.

The product managers must be specially trained not to interfere with the DRG delivery. It is the marketing responsibility to increase the number of high contribution margin DRG admissions.

MODERATE AND LOW CONTRIBUTION DRGs

This list of DRGs in a hospital may be lengthy. One should not be surprised if it is the longest of the four lists being suggested here. In the preceeding chapter, the reader should have gotten a sound idea of how individual physician practice affects the specific DRG. The concentration in this list should be on those physicians who order tests and drugs and procedures above the average number.

Bringing an individual physician closer to the average of colleagues in a specific DRG should not be difficult. For example: If a physician orders six X-ray examinations under DRG #243 (medical back problems) and other physicians order three X-rays under the same DRG, an explanation of what colleagues are doing and what the averages are may be enough to encourage a change in orders.

In the limited field trials with physicians, when the goal is getting them to change their practice pattern under specific DRGs, we have found that many physicians who see colleagues' patterns quickly try to conform to the average. True, some claim their patients are "sicker" and require additional testing and additional procedures. A patient acuity system will go far in validating (or refuting) this claim. Most physicians have simply had little communication from the hospital concerning their individual performances under specific DRGs. They seem to welcome the discussions to learn how they are performing differently from their colleagues.

Again, the product manager concept should be applied here. The choice of these product managers should be carefully considered for they will be in the forefront of medical practice change and that will take a certain personality type.

Make no mistake. As DRGs are moved from the moderate/low contribution margin list to the high contribution margin list, a major shift occurs in the hospital. The DRGs in both categories become the major line of product the individual hospital produces for the community and the medical staff soon become attuned to what products the hospital produces best. A major break-through in community perception will occur.

BELOW-POTENTIAL CONTRIBUTION DRGS

A long list for most hospitals will be those DRGs that have below-potential contribution margin for the institution. The marketer should understand that these may have high visibility factor, have major public relations value, or address a broad community need. They may be offered to fulfill a mission. They should not, therefore, be discarded by the marketer as worthless.

Take for example a hospital with the only approved burn unit in its area. The unit, from a strict contribution margin viewpoint, may take heavy toll on hospital resources. On the other hand, the public relations value, or program of support for the unit by firefighters in the area, or a major donor who gives generously to the unit, may dictate the need for retention and significant marketing of the financial "loser."

Others in this category may have the same reason for being retained and marketed. The marketing people will do well to have someone other than themselves — the administration, the board, or others — determine if one of these loser services should be discontinued or de-marketed to the point of nonexistence for the hospital.

Moving one of the below-potential DRGs to the break-even and profit making categories can be a mammoth undertaking. Much effort and many re-

sources can be put into the conversion without success. Marketers and administrators should know
clearly the risks of these attempts. Few have suc-
ceeded.

Bear in mind that "below-potential" is principally
a relative term. Relative to the higher contribution
margins presented by other DRGs, there is an opportunity cost associated with policy to capture volume
and share in those DRGs, diverting resources to the
"below-potential" group.

CHAPTER 5

Marketing by DRG: Physicians are key

In the DRG context, marketing means generating more patients within a specific DRG to reach an organizational objective (profit, market share, community need, etc.). How is it done? One fundamental way: by physicians admitting patients to the hospital. This chapter deals with a special kind of promotion — physician-related.[1]

The question of which physicians admit which DRGs must be answered first. The information needed by the marketer is the name (or code designation) of the physician and the DRGs his or her patients produce in the hospital. In a large hospital, the

[1] In an increasing number of markets, the physicians' leverage in directing patients has been diluted by PPOs, HMOs, pre-admission certification and other changes. These only change the form, not the substance, of patient origin. You can discover patient origins, whatever their manifestations, and apply the advice of this chapter.

computer should be capable of producing a report like this and in many instances already does. In a smaller hospital, the report may need to be generated by hand in the medical records department. The marketer is unable to promote particular DRGs without knowing which physicians now produce what in the hospital.

We have suggested that the marketer can view the DRGs in a given hospital as products. The challenge is to manage these products, increasing volume and share in some areas, and de-marketing in others.

Now the marketer has in hand the products (DRGs) and the producer (doctor) of each product.

The contention here is that simply sharing the information with the physician will likely produce more DRG admissions. That the physicians involved are taking some of their patients with the specific DRG to other hospitals may or may not be a real concern. If they are, the story you have to tell them is a strong one: your hospital produces the DRG more efficiently and this alone should persuade physicians to use your hospital for the DRG involved.

In those cases where a physician brings to your hospital a broad band of DRGs, the problem becomes one of first, reinforcing admitting patterns and second, generating more patients that have the possibility of producing a targeted DRG. This means enhancing the practice — getting more patients for that physician. The good healthcare marketers know how to do this or where to get the professional help to do this. Without question, the physicians will welcome such assistance.

Some hospitals have developed sophisticated programs for their physicians. They employ people who visit doctor's offices in much the same way as pharmaceutical company detail persons do. In the hospital sales forces that are now emerging, these people may act as trouble shooters for the physician's staff. They clarify hospital problems physicians may have, such as admitting difficulties, test results, information about patients, and others. In some instances, too, these people are experts in office procedures and help the physician with office management situations.

These same physician relations people should be capable of dealing with the DRG promotional efforts. They should be capable of explaining to the physicians their DRG performance in the hospital generally (they really don't know this unless the hospital shares the information it has with them) and specifically about the profitable DRGs they are producing.

Sharing the DRG information with the physician through a hospital physician relations person may require a specific orientation to the physician's practice. For instance, physician "A" has an aging practice, and DRG #138 is a disease limited to 70+ (or comorbidity and complications). The physician relations person and the physician need to understand that the hospital produces this DRG more efficiently than others. The effect of that information on the physician will in itself be useful and may result in more DRG #138 admissions. The physician's performance with admissions under that DRG will prove or disprove the suggestion being made here.

Dr. "B" may have a younger patient profile. Those diagnoses that are targeted by the hospital which fit into younger age-groups should be stressed.

Again, so that the point is made solidly, DRGs' contribution margins measure efficiency and not quality. It does not follow that a high contribution margin DRG is a quality performance by the institution.

It would be unusual to find a physician on your staff who produces DRG admissions that are always high contribution margin. Medical practices just aren't structured that way. But in those conversations with individual physicians about high contribution margin DRGs, it is also important to discuss the moderate or below-potential DRGs and what can be done about them.

Viewing the DRG as a product produced by the hospital brings into focus the very essence of the hospital's existence. Sharing this with the physicians who are really responsible for the admissions brings them to the heart of the matter. If the income for all healthcare providers is to be based on individual diagnoses of patient, then it is to the physician's advantage to know how DRGs affect the hospital because it's in his or her interest to see the hospital survive.

Viewing the DRG by contribution margin can also assist the marketer (or whoever else has the responsibility) in recruiting new physicians to the hospital staff. On the down side, recruiting a doctor whose practice will dictate low contribution margin DRGs for the hospital would be a tactical error. But recruiting physicians who are likely to produce high contribution margin DRGs could lead to greater market strength.

The point being made here bears elaboration. Most hospitals view the recruitment of physicians in the gross sense: "We need three family practitioners, two general surgeons, a pediatrician, and four internists" is the usual manner in which physician needs are perceived and voiced. A recruitment program is designed to bring physicians to your staff who produce DRGs in which the hospital wants to build a market position.

For physicians who have a practice either in your community or elsewhere, discovering the DRGs he or she produces can be a simple matter. Reviewing patient charts is one way; determining average age of patient is another; specialty of the physician is still another determinant. Existing practices can produce DRG equivalents with some digging and research into the practice. One important hint: physicians often keep a separate record of hospitalized patients and their diagnoses on an annual basis. Ask the physician to share this since it is often an easy matter to convert those diagnoses into DRGs.

The major issue here surrounds the physician who begins to practice in your area right out of a residency. What DRGs will be produced? Family practitioners are the biggest problem. A new family practitioner will usually take any patient no matter that patient's age or physical condition. If the new practitioner's office is in a location with young families surrounding it, one can bet the practice will have a low age profile. And he or she should be encouraged to attract those young families and individuals.

Family practitioners are in such heavy demand by most hospitals it would be foolhardy to detail any warnings of how their practice might alter DRG patterns. One should carefully monitor, however, the new family practitioner's admissions for DRG variables.

Internal medicine practitioners are the next toughest to recruit to a DRG system. These physicians are usually non-specialists, but some internists do have specialty areas: liver, blood system, and other specific interests. Predicting their DRG admissions to the hospital may be difficult.

Finding those doctors who produce the DRGs in which the hospital wants to build volume may not be a simple process either.

Surgeons and sub-specialists are the easiest to match to DRGs. One can easily determine what DRGs these doctors produce and matching those to profitability is the name of the game. The difficulty is growing and nurturing the primary care network from which the specialists draw referrals.

SUMMARY

The hospital marketer's promotion applications for DRGs should be clear. For the first time, the DRG designations and the income from them says clearly what products the hospital produces. No matter how it happened, the profitable DRG speaks clearly to the point of what diagnoses the hospital has mastered from a perspective of efficiency. The hospital industry has never had a measurement of product like this before.

The promotional efforts regarding DRGs lead to the physician's office for the marketer. That's where the DRG happens or doesn't happen. Not with a newspaper advertisement, a radio commercial or through a brochure. The effort begins with an eyeball to eyeball discussion with the individual physician. It can be supported with media. Maybe. It ends when the physician understands the DRG implications and admits more potential profit-makers to your hospital.

A case example

Having identified the marketing poten-
tial of DRGs, and the preferred method for ascertain-
ing cost, it is now possible to use a case study to
clarify the concrete marketing opportunities. In this
chapter, we will use a specific DRG and trace, from
research to product management the main marketing
issues.

DRG 127 is heart failure and shock, the national
number one DRG. For this reason, we expect it to be
of keen interest to most hospital CEOs and marketing
officers, since probability suggests it will be the number one (or nearly so) DRG at most facilities.

We begin by researching basic information from
one hospital which shows us the following:

DRG 127

Total Discharges, 1984	449	
Per cent of all discharges, 1984	3.9	
Rank among all DRGs	1	
By Payor:		
Medicare (number, per cent of all DRG 127 discharges)	403	89.7
Blue Cross	9	2.0
Medicaid	13	2.8
Commercial Carriers	24	5.3*
Total Gross Revenue, 1984	$2,100,422	

*Does not add to 100 because of rounding

This broad overview identifies the importance of this DRG to the facility. At 449 discharges, it is approximately 42 per cent more than the number two DRG. Using insurance carriers as a proxy for age, we note that 90 per cent of the volume depends upon patients over 65 years old, and that only 10 per cent comes from the under 65 market.

The next step is to identify the variable cost of DRG 127. As noted, this is a difficult yet crucial step. Observation within the facility, however, demonstrates that the variable cost is approximately $1450, 31 per cent of the DRG rate of $4678, composed of the following key resource areas:

- General central supply

- Emergency department supply

- Imaging services (echocardiogram, nuclear scans, X-rays)

- Laboratory chemistry
- Pharmaceuticals
- Miscellaneous (food service, linens, etc.)

This leaves a contribution margin of $3,228.

Next, we observed the pattern of seasonality for DRG 127.

	1984	1983
January	26	38
February	45	49
March	51	38
April	42	44
May	56	34
June	28	24
July	34	34
August	31	34
September	31	35
October	34	38
November	32	35
December	39	46
	449	449

The trend indicates that the spring months (Feb-May) generate the significant volumes. In 1984, they accounted for 43.2 per cent of all discharges, in 1983,

36.7 per cent. Both of these are higher than any other four month period of the year, and the 33 per cent expected distribution. Admissions traced to physicians reveal the leaders. Care must be taken here, however, since some of the leading physicians are cardiologists. Our desire is to trace the patient origin to the primary care physician. While such information is difficult to accurately secure, insights can often be gained from emergency department preference cards, medical records, and direct inquiry of the specialist.

Having identified a major DRG, its variable cost, contribution margin, frequency, seasonality and source by physician, we can turn beyond the institution to the market. The first effort is to determine market size, and subsequently market share.

Typically, there is no sure way to collect market size and share data. In this case, however, a computer-based market size estimator was purchased. It predicted the frequency of DRG by zip code, and the hospital compared these estimates to its experience.

	1984			1983		
	Hosp. (A)[1]	Market (E)[2]	Share (E) (per cent)	Hosp. (A)	Market (E)	Share (E) (per cent)
ZIP CODE 1	317	610	51	299	636	47
ZIP CODE 2	100	588	17	112	622	18
ZIP CODE 3	38	152	25	38	158	24
TOTAL	449	1350	33.2	449	1416	31.7

1: A = actual
2: E = estimate

The hospital is located in zip code 1, which is the most heavily populated. Zip code 2 is convenient to the hospital and other facilities. Zip code 3 is a remote area of relatively sparse population, equally inconvenient to all hospitals. Zip code 1 is also somewhat disproportionately old —14 per cent age 65 +. Further, the market decline between 1983 and 1984 was expected, given reimbursement pressures.

In this case, we can see that several things are occurring. Market share in zip code 1 is up significantly. The share in zip code 3 is holding its own. The share in zip code 2 looks passable, but the decline in cases is material.

Certain of these may have been attributable to management. The overall share increase may result from a new group of emergency room physicians who started in 1984. Several life squad marketing promotions were undertaken. Upon investigation, it was learned that a competing hospital placed a cardiology office in zip code 2 in mid-1984, which is suspected for the decline there. The suspicion was corroborated by a hospital physician who, though his office was in zip code 1, drew patients from zip code 2.

With this information management assessed its situation. It had a commanding relative market share in zip code 1, estimating its competitors to have only fragmented penetration. In zip code 2, it had the number 2 market share, behind hospital B, and hospital C had placed the new physician in the zip code. In zip code 3, it had equal share with hospital B, the balance being fragmented. Its posture with life squads was improving.

Some obstacles to growth were identified, however. It was clear that no more hospitals would be licensed to perform cardiac catheterization. It was also clear that the younger heart attack patients were not depending upon the hospital. This, it was discovered, owed to the referral pattern of a major family practice group in zip code 2 but not on the hospital staff which sent cardiology referrals elsewhere. This group had young patient population and should have sent more patients. Finally, it was unlikely that one of the leading admitters could get his costs under control.

All in all, this record was good, given that the hospital did not have equipment or licenses for cardiac catheterization, or coronary bypass surgery. Its services were limited to general cardiac care.

Given the facts, the hospital plotted a course of action. Its goal was to increase DRG 127 referrals as follows:

	1984 (A)[1]	1985 (G)[2]
ZIP CODE 1	311 / 51 per cent	329 / 54 per cent
ZIP CODE 2	100 / 17 per cent	200 / 34 per cent
ZIP CODE 3	38 / 25 per cent	43 / 28 per cent
	449 = 33.2 per cent	572 = 42.3 per cent

1: A = actual, number/share
2: G = goal, number/share

Management made the following analysis, knowing the DRG rate was not going to change in 1985:

1984: 449 @ \$4678 = \$2,100,422
1985: 572 @ \$4678 = \$2,675,816

Variable costs were expected to increase by 5 per cent to \$1281, and pending an actual costing, a conservative 7 per cent increase was being used ($1551). This left a contribution margin of $3127.

The 1984 total contribution was:
$$449 \times \$3,227.82 = \$1,449,291$$

The projected 1985 total contribution is: $572 \times \$3,127 = \$1,788,644$ which would present a $339,353 increase in contribution margin. Therefore, management set the marketing budget at $50,000 for DRG 127 for 1985, in the hope that it would generate a net, post-marketing contribution of $289,353.

Having constructed a meaningful set of data, the marketing option emerged clearly. Among the programs which were considered by this facility, singly and in combination:

- equipment/rent/income subsidy to cardiologist in zip code 2
- intensified life squad effort
- change in cardiology call schedule
- change in credentialing within cardiology department
- additional nurse/technician/physician training in cardiology issues
- enhanced cardiac rehabilitation services
- promotional/public relations spotlighting of selected cardiologists
- continuing education programs for top-admitting physician in each DRG

The central point is simple. Having defined the product (DRG 127) it is now relatively simple (and much simpler than before) to construct a marketing problem and formulate a program to solve it. Now, management can evaluate a product according to the following basic checklist.

PRICE:
competitive
high (skimming)
medium
low (penetration)
"milking"
per cent of self-pay patients
regulated
capitated
volatile
stable
public perception
perceived value

PRODUCT:
life cycle
introductory ⎫ time
growth ⎪ remaining
maturity ⎬ in each
decline ⎭ phase

Ansoff's Matrix:

Growth

		Hi	Low
Share	Hi	Star	Cash Cow
	Low	Problem Child	Dog

differential advantage
market need
market size, rate of increase/
    decrease
technologic risk
cost structure
        labor/capital intensity
effect on other products
degree of management
    control
competition
market share
relative market share
equipment
hospital-based physicians
customer base profile

PROMOTION: personal selling
advertising
publicity
internal communications
seminars/continuing
    education
incentives
direct mail
equipment purchases for
    physicians
physician recruitment

DISTRIBUTION: physicians   businesses
    on-staff loyal   other
    on-staff splitters   hospitals
    on-staff inactive   schools
    off-staff targeted
    off-staff not targeted

                        call lists
                        referral patterns
                   HMOs
                   nursing homes
                   life squads/police
                        walk-in

RESEARCH: growth potential
                   changes in market need,
                        size, taste, frequency
                        of purchase, etc.
                   technological replacement/
                        displacement
                             hardware
                             knowledge

To highlight this checklist, here are some examples within specific categories.

PRICE: A hospital could face volatile commercial market prices for a DRG, from PPOs, HMOs, etc., but have regulated prices for Medicare. In this situation, it could elect to remain high price to avoid the volatility or enter the fray.

PRODUCT: A hospital had a star product, but it owed 80 per cent of its stardom to a single physician, 67 years old in solo practice.

PROMOTION: To encourage a young physician to establish a practice, the hospital guaranteed certain debts and made other incentives available.

DISTRIBUTION: A hospital knew that its future depended upon changing the referral patterns of several physicians, and it allocated funds to alter those patterns.

CHAPTER 7

Clustering DRGs

In some circumstances, looking at individual DRGs can be misleading, in that it won't tell the entire story. This is particularly true with those DRG pairs and triads where the distinctions are based upon age and/or comorbidity and complications. The balance being sought in this pursuit is between too fine a measure (DRG) and too gross a measure (MDC) of activity.

A good example is the previous chapter with its assessment of DRG 127. The marketing plan prescribed has a vulnerability which owes to DRG construction, but it's a vulnerability of less importance — in some cases. DRG 127 is gaining a reputation as a catch-all DRG, used in large measure for patients who die of "old age." Therefore, one wouldn't really attempt to build a business in DRG 127. One would build a business in treating a group of related cardiac diseases and disorders. DRG 127 would likely increase as a by-product of some success. The vulnerability? In the absence of other cardiac DRGs, DRG 127 would not, solely, in all likelihood, be subject to increase.

So, clustering the major DRGs within an MDC allows the marketer to discover several things. First, it demonstrates the dispersion of case types within the MDC. Second, it can be used to focus on different physician patterns. Third, it can be used to highlight the proportion of medical and surgical products in the facility.

The following tables will guide us through this discussion. Table I shows Top 10 DRGs in one hospital; Table II shows Top 10 MDCs; Table III shows Top 8 DRG Clusters. (There are only 8 because the clustering brought clearer focus to the effort.)

TABLE I

TOP 10 DRGs

DRG	DESCRIPTION	# DISCHARGES PER YEAR
127	Heart Failure, Shock	449
243	Medical Back Problems	395
182	Esophagitis, Gastroenteritis, Misc. Digestive Disorders, 69 + C/C	291
140	Angina Pectoris	275
039	Lens Procedures	271
183	Esophagitis, Gastroenteritis, Misc. Digestive Disorders, 69–W/O C/C	243
˙089	Simple Pneumonia + Pleurisy, 69+ C/C	218
014	Specific CV Disorders Except TIA	203
088	Chronic Obstructive Pulmonary Disease (C.O.P.D.)	169
169	Procedures of Mouth 69–W/O C/C	163

Note: W/O = without
C/C = complication and/or comorbidity
+ = years or older
- = years or younger

TABLE II

TOP 10 MDCs

MDC	DESCRIPTION	# DISCHARGES
5	Diseases & Disorders of the Circulatory System	1921
6	Diseases & Disorders of the Digestive System	1889
8	Disease of the Musculoskeletal System and Connective Tissue	1715
4	Diseases & Disorders of the Respiratory System	1143
1	Diseases & Disorders of the Nervous System	852
11	Diseases & Disorders of the Kidney & Urinary Tract	617
7	Diseases & Disorders of the Hepatobiliary System & Pancreas	499
3	Diseases & Disorders of the Ear, Nose & Throat	928
9	Diseases & Disorders of the Skin, Subcutaneous Tissue & Breast	416
13	Diseases & Disorders of the Female Reproductive System	354

TABLE III

TOP 8 DRG

CLUSTERS

MDC	DESCRIPTION	DRG	# DISCHARGES	
5	Circulatory	121	81	
		122	135	
		123	44	
		127	449	
		138	151	
		139	72	
		140	275	1207
6	Digestive	148	115	
		149	15	
		161	59	
		162	135	
		168	18	
		169	163	
		182	291	
		183	243	
		174	100	1039
8	Musculoskeletal/ Connective	209	108	
		210	109	
		214	30	
		215	144	
		243	395	786
4	Respiratory	88	169	
		89	218	
		96	129	
		97	73	
		75	84	
		76	35	708

TABLE III (Continued)

TOP 8 DRG

CLUSTERS

MDC	DESCRIPTION	DRG	# DISCHARGES	
1	Nervous	5	49	
		14	203	
		15	145	397
11	Kidney/	320	100	
	Urinary Tract	31	48	
		323	42	
		324	127	
		325	18	
		326	11	346
7	Hepatobiliary/	195	29	
	Pancreas	196	7	
		197	116	
		198	93	245
10	Endocrine/	294	140	
	Nutritional/	295	20	160
	Metabolic			

The leading MDC — number 5, Circulatory disorders — accounted for 1921 discharges in a specific period. There are 43 DRGs in MDC 5 and one question would be — What is the dispersion of the 1921 cases across the 43 DRGs? We begin by looking at the proportion of DRGs available within the institution. DRG 103 — heart transplant — is not offered, and neither are several others. This facility performed cases in 38 of the 43 DRGs.

A review of cases in MDC 5 showed the majority of effort placed in seven DRGs. These seven accounted for 1,207, or 63 per cent of the 1921 discharges. 18.4 per cent of the DRGs in this MDC generated 63 per cent of the discharges.

This knowledge can be used to focus any aspect of the marketing effort. For example, in MDC 5, the seven main DRGs are as follows:

121	Circulatory Disorders W/ AMI & CV Complic.-Disch. Alive	81
122	Circulatory Disorders W/ AMI & W/O Complic.-Disch. Alive	135
123	Circulatory Disorders W/ AMI Expired	44
127	Heart Failure & Shock	449
138	Cardiac Arrhythmia & Conduction Disorders 70 + , C/C	151
139	Cardiac Arrhythmia & Conduction Disorders 70 – W/O CC	72
140	Angina	275

TOTAL = 1207
per cent of MDC = 63
MDC 5 = DRG 103 – 145 Incl. = 43
7/38 = 18.4 per cent

Note: AMI = Acute Myocardial Infarction
CV = Cardiovascular

There are essentially four clusters: 121-3, 127, 138-9 and 140. (140 is separate since angina doesn't pertain to the preceding arrhythmia DRGs.) Let's look more closely at the 121-3 cluster.

Of immediate interest are the physicians who generated these admissions. Thirty-six physicians discharged 81 patients under DRG 121. Forty-three physicians discharged 135 patients under DRG 122. Twenty-five physicians discharged 44 patients under DRG 123. Of course, most of those physicians appear in all three DRGs. Surprisingly, however, their rankings according to several variables are very different.

The leading discharger under DRG 121 was Dr. Able with six over the period of one year. Nine of the 36 physicians (one quarter) discharged only one patient under this DRG. Dr. Able discharged five patients under DRG 122, half the total of the leader in that DRG, Dr. Baker. Dr. Baker, by the way, was one of the nine who admitted only one patient under DRG 121. Neither physician figured significantly under DRG 123 — where we might have expected an appearance by Dr. Able since it appears his patient population is sicker. DRG 123 was led by Dr. Carter, who had five of the 44 discharges. Dr. Carter, however, in contrast to Drs. Able and Baker, was a cardiologist.

What are the marketing implications? Well, there are several. Dr. Able (an internist) is presumed to have a significantly older patient population, since he dominates a DRG wherein 61 of 81 discharges were Medicare. Yet he holds very few discharges in DRG 122, wherein 65 of 135 admissions were Medicare, the balance Blue Cross and commercial insurers. Likewise, we presume Dr. Baker has a younger patient population. Who cares? The marketer who wants to help physicians, that's who. Perhaps Dr. Able is concerned about his aging patient population. Or, worse yet, has never given it a thought. The hospital can intercede to help him get the target market he wants. Perhaps Dr. Baker wants to expand her practice and is willing to absorb some older patients. The hospital, again, can arrange medical directorships of nursing homes, for example, to bolster the physician and the facility.

DOCTOR RANK IN EACH DRG/CLUSTER BY NUMBER OF DISCHARGES

| | A | | | B | C | | D |
	121	122	123	129	138	139	140
Able	1	5	3/3T	3	4	18	3
Baker	26	1	3/3T	1	4	3/2T	2
Carter	11	2	1/1	33	10	1/1T	4
Door	3	2	7/2	29	7	4 5T	10
Eagle	7	23	–	2	10	18	30
Foster	–	4	2/5	38	19	2 5T	10
Green	3	23	–	3	1	10 1T	34
Hue	11	9	–	20	2	5 1T	5
Idle	11	15	–	20	3	10 5T	26
James	11	9	–	7	7	–	1

The wide dispersion of discharges across so many physicians reveals an interesting insulating property. The hospital doesn't depend heavily on one or two physicians or groups for all of its discharges in this cluster. Sixty different physicians are involved. Again, from a marketing viewpoint this fact can be undesirable. To begin, or upgrade, a cardiology program might present a great opportunity with a broad base of physician support. Conversely, the lack of a single expert leader could make such a program very difficult to develop. However, to recruit such an expert is risky only to the extent that the group is alienated, given the broad dispersion of discharging physicians.

With respect to discharges, it tends to be true that the overall leaders appear frequently as leaders within particular DRGs, particularly in medicine (as opposed to surgery). That this is not categorically true, however, presents opportunities to build market share.

A final example about discharges. As noted, DRGs 182 and 183 are major lines for this facility. MDC 6, wherein these lie, is the number 2 MDC with 1889 discharges. DRGs 182 and 183 accounted for 543, or 28 per cent of them. An investigation into the leading physicians was revealing. The top five physicians in each DRG were completely different. Remember, only age and/or CC separate these DRGs. In fact, the top-ranked physician in DRG 183, with 14 discharges, ranked 44th in DRG 182.

This analysis clearly demonstrated that certain physicians had older populations composing their practices, and others had younger populations. This confirmed other indicators already available, of course. But this facility wanted to build non-Medicare endoscopy volume. Without this information, it would have sought volume among all 10 physicians, with young and old patients alike. Now, it could target five physicians, expending half the effort, and getting equal or better results.

How did the physicians compare on costs? In DRG 121, because so many physicians had only one discharge, it's difficult to assess. The average variable cost for all 81 cases was about $4000. The highest cost physician had two cases which averaged about $10,000, with an-over-30 day LOS. He didn't discharge any patients under DRGs 122 or 123, but he did under 127, 138 and 140. Under 127 his costs were well above the mean, but well lower than the mean for 138 and 140. Closer scrutiny would show if he had some difficult cases, or if he was a high cost physician for DRG 121.

Interestingly, Dr. Able was well above the mean for average length of stay and costs for DRG 121, where he was the leader, and 122. He was above the mean for 127, below for 138, above for 139 and 140. Of greatest concern is high volume, high cost pattern in DRG 121. A marketer would be slow to shunt patients his way until his costs more nearly aligned with the average. Dr. Baker was in sharp contrast, consistently running her costs at about 80 per cent of the average for each DRG.

PROPORTION OF MEDICAL & SURGICAL ACTIVITY

Most facilities aim for a blend of medical and surgical activity. DRGs can give a more precise indication of this blend than the customary measures of total admissions by surgeons vs. medical physicians or surgical revenue vs. medical revenue.

In this institution, it was believed that there was an approximately 50/50 ratio of surgical and medical activity. Tabulating surgical DRGs and medical DRGs proved the activity differently. Only 37.5 per cent of all discharges for the year were in surgical DRGs. In the top eight clustering, the proportion dropped to 26.8 per cent. In two of the top three clusters — respiratory and circulatory, which accounted for 1796 discharges — there were no surgical DRGs.

For the marketing manager, the message was clear; the hospital needed surgeons to whom its primary care physicians would refer. Closer study would reveal the type of surgeon needed, but this first blush analysis suggested vascular, thoracic and general surgery.

A summary view of the different DRGs and clusters is revealing. The table lists some key physicians and pertinent associated data.

This table demonstrates that individual physician rankings differ considerably. Dr. Baker leads in discharges with 71, her next nearest colleague being Dr. Able with 53. Neither is a cardiologist. The rest are in a pack at about 38. As one might expect, Drs. Baker and Able were in the top six dischargers.

Organizing for marketing DRGs

DRGs present an opportunity to more fully install a marketing structure in the hospital. For all of the discussion about hospital marketing over the past several years, very few hospitals (perhaps none) are genuinely market-oriented at all levels of management, let alone throughout the organization. The ideal is to have line managers who, when confronted with market shifts or presented market data, make prompt, accurate adjustments. The typical reply, we all know, is "our employees couldn't adjust" or "let's get a committee to look at it" or the classic "that's not the way it's done around here."

We were told of a line manager in a large department who was listening to a summary of recent market research findings. The researcher said one outpatient preference is to have the test at the appointed time. The manager laughed aloud and said, "You just don't understand the way we do things around here." We need to present new career options to these kinds of managers.

If you want to have a dramatic increase in the marketability of hospital services, all you have to do is listen. A reputation of doing the best job you can of getting patients in and out on time, with a minimum of waiting between tests, will mean an increase in business for the hospital. It's that simple.

Under the present system of hospital management, the total service rendered is sometimes little more than a disjointed sequence of events. Yes, there may be "coordination" among departments, but it's typically for their convenience, not the physician's and almost certainly not the patient's. So the logical marketing goal is to instill marketing values in the guiding precepts of line managers; to distance ourselves from this notion that "Marketing is *someone else's* job."

It's a safe bet we're never going to reach this ideal. The problems of non-healthcare companies reaching this ideal are well known, and they often operate in vastly less complex environments than ours. The question becomes, then, what sort of management structure will increase market sensitivity? The answer will depend upon the specific circumstances of each facility, but we're able to predict a generic model we think will become popular over the next several years.

MODEL MANAGEMENT STRUCTURES

The present structure for hospitals runs a long spectrum. Most are a *functional* marketing organization: a marketing vice president to whom advertising, public relations, sales and planning divisions report. It is a workable organizational structure when the organization sells a single product or highly similar group of products. But a central point of this book is that DRGs can be used to demonstrate how very different some of those products are. The functional system presents severe limitations, not the least of which is having the marketing division learn the host of different technical issues sufficiently to make reasonable recommendations. One day you may be faced with a marketing issue in alcohol rehabilitation, and the next day neurosurgery.

FUNCTIONAL MARKETING STRUCTURE

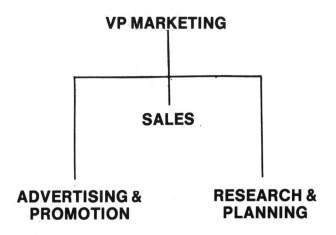

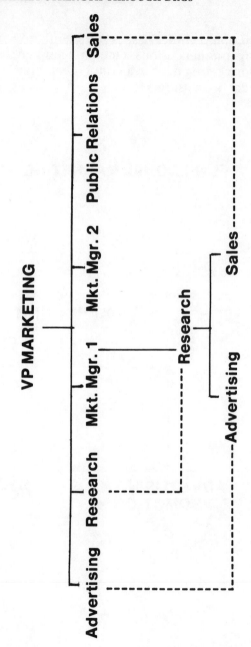

MARKET-ORIENTED STRUCTURE

Another option is a market-oriented structure, and in a limited sense this structure has evolved in some hospitals. In this case, a manager is given responsibility for managing a group of products targeted toward a specific market. The closest hospitals come to this is a vice president who focuses on medical staff (a market) and one who focuses on patients (a market). One could suggest a structure whereby a manager handles the Medicare market, another handles the HMO market, another the Blue Cross market, another the commercial insurance market, and another the private pay market. We can envision some markets where the logic of such a structure is compelling, but the mechanics of patient care could be overwhelming. We would emphasize, however, that as different payors specify different coverages and impose utilization control and so forth — which means that they are buying different products — there is a significant problem for hospitals which this structure might address.

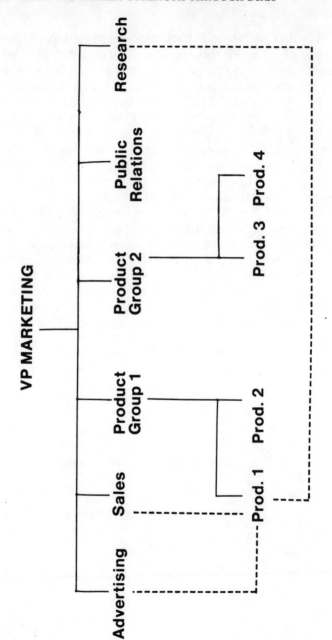

Some drawbacks of this system include its redundancy, the accompanying expense, and its elaborateness. It can become cumbersome as market managers tug at the organization for resources. And without careful coordination conflicting goals, with programs and product offerings at cross purposes, will result.

Our preference for a product-oriented system is not without reservation, but it's the best available option despite its flaws. In this structure the marketing VP preserves certain functional specialties, but individuals are given specific responsibilities for specific products (in our case, DRGs). The traditional form is as shown.

141690

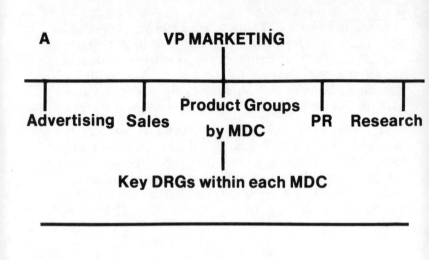

A **VP MARKETING**

Advertising   Sales   Product Groups by MDC   PR   Research

Key DRGs within each MDC

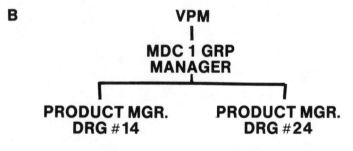

B VPM

MDC 1 GRP MANAGER

PRODUCT MGR. DRG #14   PRODUCT MGR. DRG #24

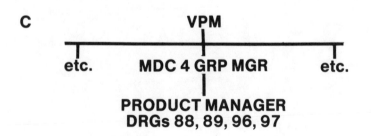

C VPM

etc.   MDC 4 GRP MGR   etc.

PRODUCT MANAGER DRGs 88, 89, 96, 97

In a hospital, size and volume will dictate the extent to which the structure need be installed. For example, volume may not support having a product manager for each of the top 10 DRGs — perhaps some can be consolidated. Some may be able to handle more than one cluster of DRGs. We've shown some alternatives.

The number of DRG clusters will, again, be a function of the organization's needs and expectations.

One of the determining factors, of course, will be the responsibilities assigned to these managers. In summary, they would be responsible for planning DRG market posture. This would embrace product, price, and promotion as predicted upon research, annual sales forecasts, product enhancements and the like. We've supplied a sample outline of an annual report each product manager would be expected to prepare and manage.

PRODUCT MANAGER
RESPONSIBILITIES
FOR DRG OR DRG CLUSTER

PRODUCT

- definition
- unique selling proposition
- equipment necessary
- expected innovations
- market niche/position

PRICE

- supporting strategy
- price sensitivity/elasticity
- discounting policy
- profit margin
- contribution margin

PROMOTION

- recommended mix:
  personal selling
  advertising
  sales promotion
  public relations

- strategy

- target audiences

DISTRIBUTION

- hospital

- physician offices

- free-standing facilities

- nursing homes

COMPETITORS AND THEIR PLANS

- a full discussion of key competitors' approaches,
  strengths, weaknesses, expected goals

SALES FORECASTS/GOALS

CAPITAL BUDGET

BUDGET OF REVENUE AND EXPENSE

PHYSICIAN RECRUITMENT/
  RETENTION PLAN

CUSTOMER PROFILE

- user-physician
- user-patients
- user-insurers
- user-businesses

EMPLOYEE TRAINING/ EDUCATION PLAN

GROWTH STRATEGY

- market penetration
- market expansion
- product enhancement

FIVE YEAR OUTLOOK AND PLAN FOR PRODUCT

- competitors
- technology
- physicians
- insurers

MARKETING INFORMATION SYSTEMS

- reports and distribution
- exception reports
- intelligence-gathering

COORDINATION WITH LINE MANAGERS

The key function is to marshall resources and information from within and without the organization to design and install a differentiated, desired product offering, appealing to physicians, HMOs, insurers, and patients. This person acts as the catalyst — some will, no doubt, say antagonist — to force market-sensitive product offerings.

The job is made extremely difficult by 1) the years of traditional techniques used in hospitals, 2) the iron-tight control over product now held by the individual department managers, 3) physician control over practice protocols, 4) regulation. These are not small differences from the consumer goods applications of product management. A pivotal difference is the ability to store product. As a service business, we can't produce and warehouse three months of X-rays, or DRG 185. It's this fact which puts so much of the product into the hands of managers and employees. Consequently, advocacy of the marketing orientation is a key duty of the product manager.

Which leads us to the single most important precedent for the successful deployment of such a system: an expressed and clearly communicated organizational goal supported by the CEO. Hospitals do this often, but almost exclusively in the arena of their building programs. "We will build a new (wing) (hospital) (clinic) (whatever)." The dollars are committed and the project is clear to everyone, if for no other reason.

A word of caution here to chief executive officers and department heads in a hospital: healthcare marketers have no "magic dust" that they spread over an organization and have miracles happen overnight. The marketing process is hard work. It takes know-how and an intelligence that understands the process and appreciates the implications of the work. Above all, the marketing process takes time. It is not the product of a day or a month or several days and several months. It is a dedication that can take years to show its value.

We have alluded to a marketing culture here and this may need some clarification. The CEO, the chief financial officer, the chief of staff, the director of nursing, the staff nurse, the director of central sterile supply — all who work in the hospital — need an appreciation of the marketing effort and its game-plan. There needs to be an environment into which the marketers ply their trade. This environment doesn't just happen; it is taught and learned. The marketing efforts that are laid on an organization without an understanding and individual relationship to that program has tough sledding and usually stalls. The effort that succeeds is the one that has full knowledge and is prepared for the effort — those are successes for the institution and for marketing. Members of the board of trustees usually understand the marketing culture. Their own enterprises engage in marketing efforts that have required the environment and culture-building discussed here. Above all, the board member who is an executive in his or her business understands full-well the seeds of marketing, the necessary plowing for those seeds, and the nurturing necessary before the crop is harvested.

CHAPTER 9

The future for DRGs

In the healthcare business, crystal-ball gazing is usually non-productive. Even the best guesses somehow never turn out the way the sooth-sayer saw them.

In the face of that unstable history, we are willing to say that DRGs are here to stay. Even if they don't stay, the marketing lessons learned in dealing with them can be valuable.

There could be variations, extensions, some contractions and some variables in the DRGs as we know them now, but conclusively there is no better basis on which hospitals are reimbursed for their care than on the structure of illness or disease. The business we are in is the attack on illness and disease—the variables of that we engage in are deviations and at best supplemental to the main thrust of our enterprise.

Prior to the DRG method of reimbursement (the "good old days" for many), hospitals controlled costs in some non-constructive way that had little effect on the bottom line. Costs were shifted regularly from this area to that area to make the prices competitive. Now the industry is faced with accurate cost finding; it is the essence of existence for an institution.

No observer of the hospital field can deny the difficulty in cost finding that is accurate. The task is difficult but essential.

Some hospitals have devised methods of billing for severity of illness or degree of illness in their nursing departments. When a patient is critically ill more nursing care is required. Conversely a patient who is not so ill requires less nursing service. Showing this differential to patients and their families is a sound step in better public acceptance of costs. The public wants to know where the money goes, and showing nursing service by degree of illness is one method for doing just that.

DRGs force the hospital into cost finding and cost controls. When specific amounts of dollars are spent for specific diagnoses, every cost analysis method needs to be applied for a true picture of the gain or loss produced by each specific DRG.

One could easily see how all payments to hospitals may become based on the DRG system. If the government, as the largest purchaser of hospital care, finds the method satisfactory, all payors will follow its lead.

That possibility should make the marketer's application of DRG product analysis and product promotion even more critical and urgent.

And consider beyond payment to a hospital by DRG from all payors payments to *physicians* by specific diagnosis. This is a real possibility for again it focuses on the disease or illness a patient presents and the work done by a physician within that diagnosis.

The possibility of a DRG method for outpatient services is just around the corner. Add the home healthcare DRG possibility, the nursing home DRG area, the office visit application, and any of the other points of entry for a patient in the healthcare system. Diagnosis is the very foundation of treatment and this irreversible fact may well dictate the payment to healthcare providers in the forseeable future.

The DRG designation may come and go, but the reality of diagnosis related reimbursement is here to stay. Any other product management alternative simply dies not make sense. There is, at present, no better method for patient classification.

It needs to be made clear beyond any doubt that while the reimbursers use a diagnosis related method for payment, the hospital marketer needs to view these as product lines. The reimburser views the method as a classification system to conserve payments or to present clear logic to their customers, subscribers, members, or congressional lawmakers. The hospital, however, needs to view these classifications as opportunities toward more sound marketing.

Bottom lines in the hospital can now be directly affected by the type of patients treated in the institution. The industry has never before had a measurement based on type of disease or illness its patients have at any given time.

One emerging solution to the problem of rising hospital costs is hospital sponsored insurance programs and other innovations alike in one dimension: they force hospitals to assume risk. Not risk in the form of Medicare's prospective payment. Rather, prepayment in the form of capitated populations, per diem payments from insurers or premium-sharing with insurers. The risk is not with individual patients, but with entire populations of people.

In many cases, this will present the final compelling incentive to cause hospitals and physicians to understand DRGs: risk pools. Risk pools are funds set aside in insurance programs to pay for patient care. To the extent that risk pools aren't drawn upon, the funds are available for distribution to the insurance plan's sponsors — frequently hospitals, physicians and insurers. Physicians and hospitals will be rewarded for managing their patients to cost-effective outcomes. This trend also underscores the marketing significance of DRGs.

Now, hospitals can bid for business by DRG. They can predict the incidence of DRGs within a given population. But to do so effectively, they'll have to look from the viewpoint presented in this book.

In the 1970's, American hospitals scoffed when a Canadian hospital specialized solely in hernia repairs and nothing else. That hospital decided to produce only its most profitable product. It could perform hernia repairs more effectively and efficiently than other hospitals and it focused on that strength.

One could conclude from what we've said about DRGs that some American hospitals should do only procedures which produce a profit. There is little chance of that happening here on a wholesale basis. Communities will require some hospitals to produce non-profitable DRGs. Factors other than profit will sustain burn units, for example.

But the notion that hospitals can provide everything for everyone will once and fo all disappear. Tertiary care centers will continue to be referral centers. Their business will increase as more and more hospitals close those units that the tertiary care centers can run more efficiently.

The marketing stance using DRGs suggested here is grounded in the notion that any given hospital does certain things better than others. Marketing those services to physicians and patients as products better produced, more effectively and more efficiently than anywhere else, is the major theme of DRG-based marketing.

It would appear that this is what the American public expects of the healthcare system: a clearer determination on behalf of that public of the best place to go for the services needed. Should anyone expect less?

Appendix: 1986 DRGs

MDC/DRG

Abbreviated Title

MDC 1: Diseases and Disorders of the Nervous System

DRG

1. Craniotomy age >17 except for trauma
2. Craniotomy for trauma age >17
3. Craniotomy age <18
4. Spinal procedures
5. Extracranial vascular procedures
6. Carpal tunnel release
7. Periph + cranial nerve + other nerv syst proc age >69 and/or C.C.
8. Periph + cranial nerve + other nerv syst proc age <70 w/o C.C.
9. Spinal disorders + injuries
10. Nervous system neoplasms age >69 and/or C.C.
11. Nervous system neoplasms age <70 w/o C.C.
12. Degenerative nervous system disorders
13. Multiple sclerosis + cerebellar ataxia
14. Specific cerebrovascular disorders except TIA
15. Transient ischemic attacks
16. Nonspecific cerebrovascular disorders with C.C.
17. Nonspecific cerebrovascular disorders w/o C.C.
18. Cranial + peripheral nerve disorders age >69 and/or C.C.
19. Cranial + peripheral nerve disorders age <70 w/o C.C.
20. Nervous system infection except viral meningitis

21	Viral meningitis
22	Hypertensive encephalopathy
23	Nontraumatic stupor + coma
24	Seizure + headache age >69 and/or C.C.
25	Seizure + headache age 18–69 w/o C.C.
26	Seizure + headache age 0–17
27	Traumatic stupor + coma, coma >1 hr
28	Traumatic stupor + coma, coma <1 hr age >69 and/or C.C.
29	Traumatic stupor + coma <1 hr age 18–69 w/o C.C.
30	Traumatic stupor + coma <1 hr age 0–17
31	Concussion age >69 and/or C.C.
32	Concussion age 18–69 w/o C.C.
33	Concussion age 0–17
34	Other disorders of nervous system age >69 and/or C.C.
35	Other disorders of nervous system age <70 w/o C.C.

MDC 2: Diseases and Disorders of the Eye

36	Retinal procedures
37	Orbital procedures
38	Primary iris procedures
39	Lens procedures
40	Extraocular procedures except orbit age >17
41	Extraocular procedures except orbit age 0–17
42	Intraocular procedures except retina, iris + lens
43	Hyphema
44	Acute major eye infections
45	Neurological eye disorders
46	Other disorders of the eye age >17 with C.C.

MDC/DRG	Abbreviated Title
47	Other disorders of the eye age >17 w/o C.C.
48	Other disorders of the eye age 0–17
MDC 3: Diseases and Disorders of the Ear, Nose and Throat	
49	Major head + neck procedures
50	Sialoadenectomy
51	Salivary gland procedures except sialoadenectomy
52	Cleft lip + palate repair
53	Sinus + mastoid procedures age >17
54	Sinus + mastoid procedures age 0–17
55	Miscellaneous ear, nose + throat procedures
56	Rhinoplasty
57	T + A proc except tonsillectomy +/or adenoidectomy only, age >17
58	T + A proc except tonsillectomy +/or adenoidectomy only, age 0–17
59	Tonsillectomy and/or adenoidectomy only age >17
60	Tonsillectomy and/or adenoidectomy only age 0–17
61	Myringotomy age >17
62	Myringotomy age 0–17
63	Other ear, nose + throat O.R. procedure
64	Ear, nose + throat malignancy
65	Dysequilibrium
66	Epistaxis
67	Epiglottitis
68	Otitis media + URI age >69 and/or C.C.
69	Otitis media + URI age 18–69 w/o C.C.
70	Otitis media + URI age 0–17
71	Laryngotracheitis
72	Nasal trauma + deformity

73	Other ear, nose + throat diagnoses age >17
74	Other ear, nose + throat diagnoses age 0–17

MDC 4: Diseases and Disorders of the Respiratory System

75	Major chest procedures
76	O.R. proc on the resp system except major chest with C.C.
77	O.R. proc on the resp system except major chest w/o C.C.
78	Pulmonary embolism
79	Respiratory infections + inflammations age >69 and/or C.C.
80	Respiratory infections + inflammations age 18–69 w/o C.C.
81	Respiratory infections + inflammations age 0–17
82	Respiratory neoplasms
83	Major chest trauma age >69 and/or C.C.
84	Major chest trauma age <70 w/o C.C.
85	Pleural effusion age >69 and/or C.C.
86	Pleural effusion age <70 w/o C.C.
87	Pulmonary edema + respiratory failure
88	Chronic obstructive pulmonary disease
89	Simple pneumonia + pleurisy age >69 and/or C.C.
90	Simple pneumonia + pleurisy age 18–69 w/o C.C.
91	Simple pneumonia + pleurisy age 0–17
92	Interstitial lung disease age >69 and/or C.C.
93	Interstitial lung disease age <70 w/o C.C.
94	Pneumothorax age >69 and/or C.C.
95	Pneumothorax age <70 w/o C.C.
96	Bronchitis + asthma age >69 and/or C.C.
97	Bronchitis + asthma age 18–69 w/o C.C.

MDC/DRG	Abbreviated Title
98	Bronchitis + asthma age 0–17
99	Respiratory signs + symptoms age >69 and/or C.C.
100	Respiratory signs + symptoms age <70 w/o C.C.
101	Other respiratory diagnoses age >69 and/or C.C.
102	Other respiratory diagnoses age <70 w/o C.C.
MDC 5: Diseases and Disorders of the Circulatory System	
103	Heart transplant
104	Cardiac valve procedure with pump + with cardiac cath
105	Cardiac valve procedure with pump and w/o cardiac cath
106	Coronary bypass with cardiac cath
107	Coronary bypass w/o cardiac cath
108	Cardiothor proc, except valve + coronary bypass, with pump
109	Cardiothoracic procedures except valve + coronary bypass, w/o pump
110	Major reconstructive vascular procedures age >69 and/or C.C.
111	Major reconstructive vascular procedures age <70 w/o C.C.
112	Vascular procedures except major reconstruction
113	Amputation for circ system disorders except upper limb + toe
114	Upper limb + toe amputation for circ system disorders
115	Permanent cardiac pacemaker implant with AMI or CHF
116	Permanent cardiac pacemaker implant w/o AMI or CHF
117	Cardiac pacemaker replace + revis exc pulse gen repl only
118	Cardiac pacemaker pulse generator replacement only
119	Vein ligation + stripping
120	Other O.R. procedures on the circulatory system
121	Circulatory disorders with AMI + c.v. comp. disch. alive
122	Circulatory disorders with AMI w/o c.v. comp. disch. alive
123	Circulatory disorders with AMI, expired

124	Circulatory disorders exc AMI, with card cath & comp diag
125	Circulatory disorders exc AMI, with card cath uncomp DX 1
126	Acute + subacute endocarditis
127	Heart failure + shock
128	Deep vein thrombophlebitis
129	Cardiac arrest
130	Peripheral vascular disorders age >69 and/or C.C.
131	Peripheral vascular disorders age <70 w/o C.C.
132	Atherosclerosis age >69 and/or C.C.
133	Atherosclerosis age <70 w/o C.C.
134	Hypertension
135	Cardiac congenital + valvular disorders age >69 and/or C.C.
136	Cardiac congenital + valvular disorders age 18–69 w/o C.C.
137	Cardiac congenital + valvular disorders age 0–17
138	Cardiac arrhythmia + conduction disorders age >69 and/or C.C.
139	Cardiac arrhythmia + conduction disorders age <70 w/o C.C.
140	Angina pectoris
141	Syncope + collapse age >69 and/or C.C.
142	Syncope + collapse age <70 w/o C.C.
143	Chest pain
144	Other circulatory diagnoses with C.C.
145	Other circulatory diagnoses w/o C.C.

MDC 6: Diseases and Disorders of the Digestive System

146	Rectal resection age >69 and/or C.C.
147	Rectal resection age <70 w/o C.C.
148	Major small + large bowel procedures age >69 and/or C.C.
149	Major small + large bowel procedures age <70 w/o C.C.

MDC/DRG	Abbreviated Title
150	Peritoneal adhesiolysis age >69 and/or C.C.
151	Peritoneal adhesiolysis age <70 w/o C.C.
152	Minor small + large bowel procedures age >69 and/or C.C.
153	Minor small + large bowel procedures age <70 w/o C.C.
154	Stomach, esophageal + duodenal procedures age >69 and/or C.C.
155	Stomach, esophageal + duodenal procedures age 18–69 w/o C.C.
156	Stomach, esophageal + duodenal procedures age 0–17
157	Anal procedures age >69 and/or C.C.
158	Anal procedures age <70 w/o C.C.
159	Hernia procedures except inguinal + femoral age >69 and/or C.C.
160	Hernia procedures except inguinal + femoral age 18–69 w/o C.C.
161	Inguinal + femoral hernia procedures age >69 and/or C.C.
162	Inguinal + femoral hernia procedures age 18–69 w/o C.C.
163	Hernia procedures age 0–17
164	Appendectomy with complicated princ. diag age >69 and/or C.C.
165	Appendectomy with complicated princ. diag age <70 w/o C.C.
166	Appendectomy w/o complicated princ. diag age >69 and/or C.C.
167	Appendectomy w/o complicated princ. diag age <70 w/o C.C.
168	Procedures on the mouth age >69 and/or C.C.
169	Procedures on the mouth age <70 w/o C.C.
170	Other digestive system procedures age >69 and/or C.C.
171	Other digestive system procedures age <70 w/o C.C.
172	Digestive malignancy age >69 and/or C.C.
173	Digestive malignancy age <70 w/o C.C.
174	G.I. hemorrhage age >69 and/or C.C.
175	G.I. hemorrhage age <70 w/o C.C.
176	Complicated peptic ulcer
177	Uncomplicated peptic ulcer >69 and/or C.C.
178	Uncomplicated peptic ulcer <70 w/o C.C.

179   Inflammatory bowel disease
180   G.I. obstruction age >69 and/or C.C.
181   G.I. obstruction age <70 w/o C.C.
182   Esophagitis, gastroent. + misc. digest. dis age >69 and/or C.C.
183   Esophagitis, gastroent. + misc. digest. dis age 18–69 w/o C.C.
184   Esophagitis, gastroenteritis + misc. digest. disorders age 0–17
185   Dental + oral dis. exc extractions + restorations, age >17
186   Dental + oral dis. exc extractions + restorations, age 0–17
187   Dental extractions + restorations
188   Other digestive system diagnoses age >69 and/or C.C.
189   Other digestive system diagnoses age 18–69 w/o C.C.
190   Other digestive system diagnoses age 0–17

MDC 7: Diseases and Disorders of the Hepatobiliary System and Pancreas

191   Major pancreas, liver + shunt procedures
192   Minor pancreas, liver + shunt procedures
193   Biliary tract proc exc tot cholecystectomy age >69 and/or C.C.
194   Biliary tract proc exc tot cholecystectomy age <70 w/o C.C.
195   Total cholecystectomy w c.d.e. age >69 and/or C.C.
196   Total cholecystectomy w c.d.e. age <70 w/o C.C.
197   Total cholecystectomy w/o c.d.e. age >69 and/or C.C.
198   Total cholecystectomy w/o c.d.e. age <70 w/o C.C.
199   Hepatobiliary diagnostic procedure for malignancy
200   Hepatobiliary diagnostic procedure for non-malignancy
201   Other hepatobiliary or pancreas O.R. procedures
202   Cirrhosis + alcoholic hepatitis
203   Malignancy of hepatobiliary system or pancreas

MDC/DRG	Abbreviated Title
204	Disorders of pancreas except malignancy
205	Disorders of liver exc malig, cirr, alc hepa age >69 and/or C.C.
206	Disorders of liver exc malig, cirr, alc hepa age <70 w/o C.C.
207	Disorders of the biliary tract age >69 and/or C.C.
208	Disorders of the biliary tract age <70 w/o C.C.
MDC 8: Diseases and Disorders of the Musculoskeletal System and Connective Tissue	
209	Major joint procedures
210	Hip + femur procedures except major joint age >69 and/or C.C.
211	Hip + femur procedures except major joint age 18–69 w/o C.C.
212	Hip + femur procedures except major joint age 0–17
213	Amputations for musculoskeletal system + conn. tissue disorders
214	Back + neck procedures age >69 and/or C.C.
215	Back + neck procedures age <70 w/o C.C.
216	Biopsies of musculoskeletal system + connective tissue
217	Wnd debrid + skn grft exc hand, for muscskseletal + conn. tiss. dis
218	Lower extrem + humer proc exc hip, foot, femur age >69 and/or C.C.
219	Lower extrem + humer proc exc hip, foot, femur age 18–69 w/o C.C.
220*	Lower extrem + humer proc exc hip, foot, femur age 0–17
221	Knee procedures age >69 and/or C.C.
222	Knee procedures age <70 w/o C.C.
223	Upper extremity proc exc humerus + hand age >69 and/or C.C.
224	Upper extremity proc exc humerus + hand age <70 w/o C.C.
225	Foot procedures
226	Soft tissue procedures age >69 and/or C.C.
227	Soft tissue procedures age <70 w/o C.C.

228 Ganglion hand procedures
229 Hand procedures except ganglion
230 Local excision + removal of int fix devices of hip + femur
231 Local excision + removal of int fix devices except hip + femur
232 Arthroscopy
233 Other musculoskelet sys + conn tiss O.R. proc age >69 and/or C.C.
234 Other musculoskelet sys + conn tiss O.R. proc age <70 w/o C.C.
235 Fractures of femur
236 Fractures of hip + pelvis
237 Sprains, strains, + dislocations of hip, pelvis + thigh
238 Osteomyelitis
239 Pathological fractures + musculoskeletal + conn. tiss. malignancy
240 Connective tissue disorders age >69 and/or C.C.
241 Connective tissue disorders age <70 w/o C.C.
242 Septic arthritis
243 Medical back problems
244 Bone diseases + septic arthropathy age >69 and/or C.C.
245 Bone diseases + septic arthropathy age <70 w/o C.C.
246 Non-specific arthropathies
247 Signs + symptoms of musculoskeletal system + conn tissue
248 Tendonitis, myositis + bursitis
249 Aftercare, musculoskeletal system + connective tissue
250 Fx, sprns, strns + disl of forearm, hand, foot age >69 and/or C.C.
251 Fx, sprns, strns + disl of forearm, hand, foot age 18–69 w/o C.C.
252 Fx, sprns, strns + disl of forearm, hand, foot age 0–17
253 Fx, sprns, strns + disl of uparm, lowleg ex foot age >69 and/or C.C.
254 Fx, sprns, strns + disl of uparm, lowleg ex foot age 18–69 w/o C.C.
255 Fx, sprns, strns + disl of uparm, lowleg ex foot age 0–17
256 Other diagnoses of musculoskeletal system + connective tissue

MDC/DRG

Abbreviated Title

MDC 9: Diseases and Disorders of the Skin, Subcutaneous Tissue and Breast

257	Total mastectomy for malignancy age >69 and/or C.C.
258	Total mastectomy for malignancy age <70 w/o C.C.
259	Subtotal mastectomy for malignancy age >69 and/or C.C.
260	Subtotal mastectomy for malignancy age <70
261	Breast proc for non-malig except biopsy + loc exc
262	Breast biopsy + local excision for non-malignancy
263	Skin grafts for skin ulcer or cellulitis age >69 and/or C.C.
264	Skin grafts for skin ulcer or cellulitis age <70 w/o C.C.
265	Skin grafts except for skin ulcer or cellulitis with C.C.
266	Skin grafts except for skin ulcer or cellulitis w/o C.C.
267	Perianal + pilonidal procedures
268	Skin, subcutaneous tissue + breast plastic procedures
269	Other skin, subcut tiss + breast O.R. proc age >69 and/or C.C.
270	Other skin, subcut tiss + breast O.R. proc age <70 w/o C.C.
271	Skin ulcers
272	Major skin disorders age >69 and/or C.C.
273	Major skin disorders age <70 w/o C.C.
274	Malignant breast disorders age >69 and/or C.C.
275	Malignant breast disorders age <70 w/o C.C.
276	Non-malignant breast disorders
277	Cellulitis age >69 and/or C.C.
278	Cellulitis age 18–69 w/o C.C.
279	Cellulitis age 0–17
280	Trauma to the skin, subcut tiss + breast age >69 and/or C.C.
281	Trauma to the skin, subcut tiss + breast age 18–69 w/o C.C.

282   Trauma to the skin, subcut tiss + breast age 0–17

283   Minor skin disorders age >69 and/or C.C.

284   Minor skin disorders age <70 w/o C.C.

MDC 10: Endocrine, Nutritional and Metabolic Diseases and Disorders

285   Amputations for endocrine, nutritional + metabolic disorders

286   Adrenal + pituitary procedures

287   Skin grafts + wound debride for endoc, nutrit + metab disorders

288   O.R. procedures for obesity

289   Parathyroid procedures

290   Thyroid procedures

291   Thyroglossal procedures

292   Other endocrine, nutrit + metab O.R. proc age >69 and/or C.C.

293   Other endocrine, nutrit + metab O.R. proc age <70 w/o C.C.

294   Diabetes age = >36

295   Diabetes age 0–35

296   Nutritional + misc. metabolic disorders age >69 and/or C.C.

297   Nutritional + misc. metabolic disorders age 18–69 w/o C.C.

298   Nutritional + misc. metabolic disorders age 0–17

299   Inborn errors of metabolism

300   Endocrine disorders age >69 and/or C.C.

301   Endocrine disorders age <70 w/o C.C.

MDC/DRG

MDC 11: Diseases and Disorders of the Kidney and Urinary Tract

Abbreviated Title

302	Kidney transplant
303	Kidney, ureter + major bladder procedure for malignancy
304	Kidney, ureter + maj bldr proc for non-malig age >69 and/or C.C.
305	Kidney, ureter + maj bldr proc for non-malig age <70 w/o C.C.
306	Prostatectomy age >69 and/or C.C.
307	Prostatectomy age <70 w/o C.C.
308	Minor bladder procedures age >69 and/or C.C.
309	Minor bladder procedures age <70 w/o C.C.
310	Transurethral procedures age >69 and/or C.C.
311	Transurethral procedures age <70 w/o C.C.
312	Urethral procedures, age >69 and/or C.C.
313	Urethral procedures, age 18–69 w/o C.C.
314	Urethral procedures, age 0–17
315	Other kidney + urinary tract O.R. procedures
316	Renal failure w/o dialysis
317	Renal failure w/dialysis
318	Kidney + urinary tract neoplasms age >69 and/or C.C.
319	Kidney + urinary tract neoplasms age <70 w/o C.C.
320	Kidney + urinary tract infections age >69 and/or C.C.
321	Kidney + urinary tract infections age 18–69 w/o C.C.
322	Kidney + urinary tract infections age 0–17
323	Urinary stones age >69 and/or C.C.
324	Urinary stones age <70 w/o C.C.
325	Kidney + urinary tract signs + symptoms age >69 and/or C.C.
326	Kidney + urinary tract signs + symptoms age 18–69 w/o C.C.
327	Kidney + urinary tract signs + symptoms age 0–17

328	Urethral stricture age >69 and/or C.C.
329	Urethral stricture age 18–69 w/o C.C.
330	Urethral stricture age 0–17
331	Other kidney + urinary tract diagnoses age >69 and/or C.C.
332	Other kidney + urinary tract diagnoses age 18–69 w/o C.C.
333	Other kidney + urinary tract diagnoses age 0–17

MDC 12: Diseases and Disorders of the Male Reproductive System

334	Major male pelvic procedures with C.C.
335	Major male pelvic procedures w/o C.C.
336	Transurethral prostatectomy age >69 and/or C.C.
337	Transurethral prostatectomy age <70 w/o C.C.
338	Testes procedures, for malignancy
339	Testes procedures, non-malignant age >17
340	Testes procedures, non-malignant age 0–17
341	Penis procedures
342	Circumcision age >17
343	Circumcision age 0–17
344	Other male reproductive system O.R. procedures for malignancy
345	Other male reproductive system O.R. proc except for malignancy
346	Malignancy, male reproductive system, age >69 and/or C.C.
347	Malignancy, male reproductive system, age <70 w/o C.C.
348	Benign prostatic hypertrophy age >69 and/or C.C.
349	Benign prostatic hypertrophy age <70 w/o C.C.
350	Inflammation of the male reproductive system
351	Sterilization, male
352	Other male reproductive system diagnoses

MDC/DRG   **Abbreviated Title**

MDC 13: Diseases and Disorders of the Female Reproductive System

353	Pelvic evisceration, radical hysterectomy + vulvectomy
354	Non-radical hysterectomy age >69 and/or C.C.
355	Non-radical hysterectomy age <70 w/o C.C.
356	Female reproductive system reconstructive procedures
357	Uterus + adenexa procedures, for malignancy
358	Uterus + adenexa proc for non-malignancy except tubal interrupt
359	Tubal interruption for non-malignancy
360	Vagina, cervix + vulva procedures
361	Laparoscopy + endoscopy (female) except tubal interruption
362	Laparoscopic tubal interruption
363	D+C, conization + radio-implant, for malignancy
364	D+C, conization except for malignancy
365	Other female reproductive system O.R. procedures
366	Malignancy, female reproductive system age >69 and/or C.C.
367	Malignancy, female reproductive system age <70 w/o C.C.
368	Infections, female reproductive system
369	Menstrual + other female reproductive system disorders

MDC 14: Pregnancy, Childbirth, and the Puerperium

370	Cesarean section with C.C.
371	Cesarean section w/o C.C.
372	Vaginal delivery with complicating diagnoses
373	Vaginal delivery w/o complicating diagnoses
374	Vaginal delivery with sterilization and/or D+C

375 Vaginal delivery with O.R. proc except steril and/or D+C
376 Postpartum diagnoses w/o O.R. procedure
377 Postpartum diagnoses with O.R. procedure
378 Ectopic pregnancy
379 Threatened abortion
380 Abortion w/o D+C
381 Abortion with D+C
382 False labor
383 Other antepartum diagnoses with medical complications
384 Other antepartum diagnoses w/o medical complications

MDC 15: Newborns and Other Neonates with Conditions Originating in the Perinatal Period

385 Neonates, died or transferred
386 Extreme immaturity, neonate
387 Prematurity w/ major problems
388 Prematurity w/o major problems
389 Full term neonate with major problems
390 Neonates with other significant problems
391 Normal newborns

MDC/DRG	Abbreviated Title
MDC 16: Diseases and Disorders of the Blood and Blood-Forming Organs and Immunological Disorders	
392	Splenectomy age >17
393	Splenectomy age 0–17
394	Other O.R. procedures of the blood + blood forming organs
395	Red blood cell disorders age >17
396	Red blood cell disorders age 0–17
397	Coagulation disorders
398	Reticuloendothelial + immunity disorders age >69 and/or C.C.
399	Reticuloendothelial + immunity disorders age <70 w/o C.C.
MDC 17: Myeloproliferative Diseases and Disorders and Poorly Differentiated Neoplasms	
400	Lymphoma or leukemia with major O.R. procedure
401	Lymphoma or leukemia with minor O.R. proc age >69 and/or C.C.
402	Lymphoma or leukemia with minor O.R. procedure age <70 w/o C.C.
403	Lymphoma or leukemia age >69 and/or C.C.
404	Lymphoma or leukemia age 18–69 w/o C.C.
405	Lymphoma or leukemia age 0–17
406	Myeloprolif disord or poorly diff neoplasm w maj O.R. proc + C.C.
407	Myeloprolif disord or poorly diff neopl w maj O.R. proc w/o C.C.
408	Myeloprolif disord or poorly diff neopl with minor O.R. proc
409	Radiotherapy

410	Chemotherapy
411	History of malignancy w/o endoscopy
412	History of malignancy with endoscopy
413	Other myeloprolif disord or poorly diff neopl DX age >69 and/or C.C.
414	Other myeloprolif disord or poorly diff neopl DX age <70 w/o C.C.

MDC 18: Infectious and Parasitic Diseases (Systemic or Un-specified Sites)

415	O.R. procedure for infectious + parasitic diseases
416	Septicemia age >17
417	Septicemia age 0–17
418	Postoperative + post-traumatic infections
419	Fever of unknown origin age >69 and/or C.C.
420	Fever of unknown origin age 18–69 w/o C.C.
421	Viral illness age >17
422	Viral illness + fever of unknown origin age 0–17
423	Other infectious + parasitic diseases diagnoses

MDC 19: Mental Diseases and Disorders

424	O.R. procedures with principal diagnosis of mental illness
425	Acute adjust react + disturbances of psychosocial dysfunction
426	Depressive neuroses
427	Neuroses except depressive
428	Disorders of personality + impulse control
429	Organic disturbances + mental retardation
430	Psychoses

MDC/DRG   **Abbreviated Title**

431   Childhood mental disorders
432   Other diagnoses of mental disorders

MDC 20: Substance Use and Substance Induced Organic Mental Disorders

433   Substance use + substance induced organic mental disorders, left AMA
434   Drug dependence
435   Drug use except dependence
436   Alcohol dependence
437   Alcohol use except dependence
438   Alcohol + substance induced organic mental syndrome

MDC 21: Injury, Poisoning and Toxic Effects of Drugs

439   Skin grafts for injuries
440   Wound debridements for injuries
441   Hand procedures for injuries
442   Other O.R. procedures for injuries age >69 and/or C.C.
443   Other O.R. procedures for injuries age <70 w/o C.C.
444   Multiple trauma age >69 and/or C.C.
445   Multiple trauma age 18–69 w/o C.C.
446   Multiple trauma age 0–17
447   Allergic reactions age >17
448   Allergic reactions age 0–17
449   Toxic effects of drugs age >69 and/or C.C.
450   Toxic effects of drugs age 18–69 w/o C.C.

451	Toxic effects of drugs age 0–17
452	Complications of treatment age >69 and/or C.C.
453	Complications of treatment age <70 w/o C.C.
454	Other injuries, poisonings + toxic eff drugs age >69 and/or C.C.
455	Other injuries, poisonings + toxic eff drugs age <70 w/o C.C.

MDC 22: Burns

456	Burns, transferred to another acute care facility
457	Extensive burns
458	Non-extensive burns with skin grafts
459	Non-extensive burns with wound debridement + O.R. proc
460	Non-extensive burns w/o O.R. procedure

MDC 23: Factors Influencing Health Status and Other Contacts with Health Services

461	O.R. proc with diagnoses of other contact with health services
462	Rehabilitation
463	Signs + symptoms with C.C.
464	Signs + symptoms w/o C.C.
465	Aftercare with history of malignancy as secondary DX
466	Aftercare w/o history of malignancy as secondary DX
467	Other factors influencing health status
468	Unrelated O.R. procedure
469	PDX invalid as discharge diagnosis
470	Ungroupable

Index

DATE DUE

DEC T 2 '87	MAY 0 7 '88		
MAR 16 1990			
Returned			
APR 13 1990			
MAY 0 4 1990			
NOV 27 1991			
V 0 8 1992			
Returned			
APR 15 1994			
Returned			
MAR 2 5 '96			
MAY 0 8 '96			
MAR 2 7 97			